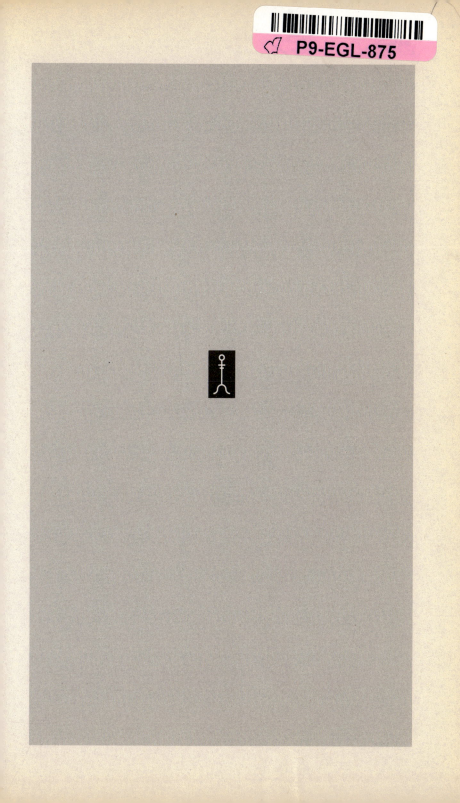

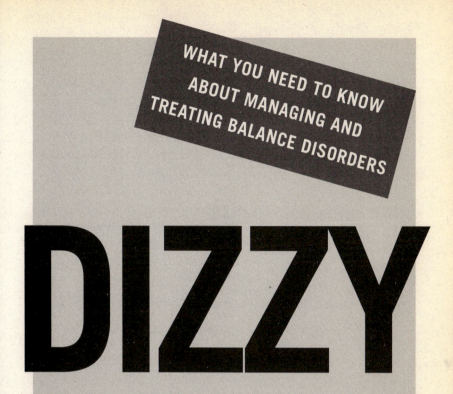

WHAT YOU NEED TO KNOW
ABOUT MANAGING AND
TREATING BALANCE DISORDERS

DIZZY

JACK J. WAZEN, M.D.

with Deborah Mitchell

A LYNN SONBERG BOOK

A Fireside Book
Published by Simon & Schuster
New York   London   Toronto   Sydney

FIRESIDE
Rockefeller Center
1230 Avenue of the Americas
New York, NY 10020

FIRESIDE and colophon are registered trademarks of Simon & Schuster, Inc.

For information about special discounts for bulk purchases, please contact
Simon & Schuster Special Sales:
1-800-456-6798 or business@simonandschuster.com

Designed by William Ruoto

Manufactured in the United States of America

5 7 9 10 8 6 4

Library of Congress Cataloging-in-Publication Data
Wazen, Jack J.
Dizzy: what you need to know about managing and treating balance
disorders / Jack J. Wazen, with Deborah Mitchell.
p. cm.
"A Lynn Sonberg book."
Includes bibliographical references and index.
1. Vestibular apparatus —Diseases. 2. Dizziness—Treatment.
3. Equilibrium (Physiology). I. Mitchell, Deborah R. II. Title.
RF260.W39   2004
617.8'82—dc22   2003061658
ISBN-13: 978-0-7432-3622-5 (Pbk)
ISBN-10:   0-7432-3622-X (Pbk)

Contents

Preface

For years I have watched people climb into the cars and seats of amusement park rides; strap themselves into whirling cups, roller coasters, and ferris wheels; and be flung screaming into the air. I've seen how some of them stagger and sway when they get off the ride and the tinge of green around their mouth. And I've noticed that some of them turn around, purchase another ticket, and stand in line again for a second ride.

As a physician who has dedicated much of my professional life to treating people who are plagued with lightheadedness, dizziness, and balance problems and whose lives can be literally turned upside down by these problems, two thoughts come into my mind as I observe these folks. One betrays my scientific leanings: Wouldn't it be interesting to enroll these people in a research study and perform various inner ear tests on them? The ride going on inside their ears is likely far more exciting (to me at least) than the one their body is involved in. The second thought is mere curiosity: Why do they do this to themselves? Do they really *want* to be dizzy and nauseous?

As medical director of the Balance Management Center at Lenox Hill Hospital in New York City, I've seen thousands of people who live in fear of dizziness and of losing their balance. I've treated hundreds of individuals, young and old, who wouldn't leave their homes because they were afraid they might have a severe attack of dizziness or lose their balance while walking up the stairs or crossing the street. I've seen many elderly people who felt isolated and frightened because they could no longer walk across a room without feeling dizzy or get up out of a chair without falling. And I've known scores of men and women who never knew when their world would, without warning, begin to swirl and spin around them. Many of these people suffered for months or even years without knowing what was wrong with them. They went from doctor to doctor looking for an explanation, and found none.

Riding a roller coaster is probably the last place on earth any of these people would want to be.

So there are two kinds of people in the world: those who think it's fun to be dizzy and those who don't. Because you've picked up this book, I'm guessing that you are in the latter category and you're looking for answers. I'm pleased to tell you, you've come to the right place.

According to the National Institutes of Health, at least 90 million Americans (42 percent of the population) will seek a doctor's care for dizziness at least once during their lifetime. And according to the Centers for Disease Control and Prevention, 4 percent of all American adults—about 10 million people—have felt dizzy or experienced poor balance within the previous three months.

Whether you're among the 90 million or the 10 million—or you know someone who is—this book can help. Chances are, you've got questions about dizziness and balance problems, and I imagine that near the top of your list are the following: Why am I dizzy? Why do I lose my balance? And, what can I do about it?

In this book, we answer these questions and many more. The bottom line is this: There are many ways to treat dizziness and balance problems, and many of them you can do at home (with prior assistance from your physician or other health-care practitioner) or, if necessary, at a balance treatment center that can offer you permanent solutions to your balance problems.

Sound too good to be true? Then consider this: 80 to 90 percent of people who have a balance disorder can be helped through balance retraining exercises, diet, medications, or, infrequently, surgery. This book tells you about these approaches, and more.

Balance disorders can affect people of any age, gender, or ethnicity, but I see them more often and with increasing frequency among older people. And as the baby boomer population ages, we can expect to see a substantial rise in the number of people with balance disturbances.

Already, more than 5 million doctor visits for dizziness or vertigo are made every year in the United States. Medical care for Americans with balance disorders is estimated to exceed $1 billion annually. And the emotional and social costs, although without a dollar figure attached to them, are staggering as well. Those costs come in the form of fear and anxiety: people afraid to leave their homes, people who can no longer work or go to school, people who must sleep sitting up because they get too dizzy when they lie down, in short, people whose lives are in turmoil.

There are literally dozens of reasons you can experience a balance problem. At the Tinnitus, Hearing and Balance Center at Columbia-Presbyterian Medical Center in New York, which I founded in the early 1990s and for which I was formerly the medical director, I had literally "seen them all." Many of the people I've seen over the years had already consulted several other doctors and walked away without a definitive diagnosis. They felt discouraged, frustrated, and worried. In fact on average, individuals who have problems with balance consult six different doctors before they are diagnosed correctly and can begin an effective treatment program. That's because few doctors, including ear-nose-throat (ENT, or otolaryngology) specialists, are well versed in balance disorders.

In fact, most ENTs are not interested in balance and tinnitus. Thus millions of Americans suffer months or even years of fear, frustration, and life-altering symptoms before they get help from a balance specialist. One of the purposes of this book is to offer you guidelines that can help you identify the cause of your dizziness so you can then work with the right specialist(s) who can ensure you get an accurate diagnosis and effective treatment, which will allow you to live your life in balance again.

Norma is one such individual whose life was dramatically changed by a balance disorder. The 33-year-old executive secretary has Ménière's disease, a condition characterized by vertigo (when it feels as if the world around you is spinning), tinnitus (ringing in the ears), and hearing loss. After battling these unexplained symptoms for more than six months and visiting several doctors who could not identify her problem, she finally found her way to my center. By that time, however, she had quit her job because daily vertigo attacks made it impossible for her to work. She was afraid to drive or to walk far from her apartment, so she spent much of her time sequestered inside.

Once we made the diagnosis, she was ready to undergo extensive rehabilitation therapy, which included exercises she did at the Balance Management Center and at home. She also took a mild sedative for a short time and switched to a low-salt diet to help maintain good inner ear fluid levels. Within two months she improved enough to return to work part-time, and after four months she was working full-time again.

For Richard, a 49-year-old general contractor, it was a more common balance problem called benign paroxysmal positional vertigo that knocked him off his feet. After suffering a blow to the head from a wooden beam carried by fellow workers, he felt momentarily stunned but was able to continue working. The next day, however, while bending over to tie his shoe, he felt violently dizzy and fell to the ground. The feeling passed after a few seconds, but in subsequent days similar movements of his head caused him to feel as if the world was spinning. Because these dizzy spells made doing his job extremely dangerous, Richard called his doctor. Fortunately, Richard's primary care physician suspected benign paroxysmal positional vertigo on the basis of his history and symptoms and referred him to us. Once we determined Richard did have benign paroxysmal positional vertigo, he was treated with special positioning maneuvers and his vertigo cleared up.

Symptoms such as vertigo, lightheadedness, nausea, tinnitus, and dizziness can happen suddenly or come on slowly. They may last for seconds or days; occur routinely or sporadically. Overall, approximately 250 different medical conditions are associated with balance problems. Thus it is easy to see how such a large number of factors can make discovering the cause of a balance problem very difficult for physicians and frustrating for both patients and their doctors.

If you're suffering that frustration, this book can help you eliminate it. Here's how.

How to Use This Book

This book is divided into three parts, each of which builds on the other. In part I, two things are important for you to remember: (1) The best antidote for frustration is knowledge and understanding, and (2) Accurate input from you about your symptoms is critical in helping your doctors make an accurate diagnosis. Therefore, in part I we arm you with the tools you need to understand what's happening to you. What does it mean to be dizzy? What is vertigo? What does it mean to lose your balance? We offer explanations and a checklist to help you identify your experiences so you can provide your doctor with the most accurate information possible.

The first steps to getting an accurate diagnosis are finding a competent health-care practitioner and undergoing initial diagnostic procedures. Thus the remainder of part I is dedicated to helping you select the right physician, discussing the importance of the dizziness questionnaire and a thorough medical history, and explaining the various procedures and tests your health-care provider may perform during his or her initial diagnostic process.

People want to understand what is happening to them—the causes, risk factors, and symptoms of their disorders—and how they can get better. So the second part of this book is a discussion of the various types of balance disorders. Each chapter covers different types of conditions that can be associated with dizziness, vertigo, and/or balance problems; how you can recognize these conditions; and what treatment options are available. You will learn, for example, the impact blood pressure or other heart-related problems have on balance, how thyroid disorders and kidney disease can make you dizzy, and which medications—over-the-counter and prescription—affect the inner ear.

In part II, you will meet people who have come to my center and hear their stories of diagnosis and successful treatment. The section ends with a discussion of the types of specialized tests and measurements that are often conducted when individuals are referred to a specialist.

People who have the flu or a mild ear infection can expect to feel lightheaded and nauseous for a day or two, and for the most part, these are temporary symptoms that go away once the infection clears. But for the millions of people who suffer with conditions characterized by chronic or intermittent dizziness, vertigo, or disequilibrium, relief is not always easy to find.

That's where this book shines. In part III, "Stop the World: Treating Balance Disorders," we offer you the tools you need to help get relief. The good news is that for the majority of people, significant relief or elimination of their symptoms is possible, using a combination of lifestyle changes, including diet, stress management, and supplements; rehabilitation exercises, which often can be done at home or on an outpatient basis; medication, if needed; and rarely, surgery, which is usually reserved for severe cases that do not respond to other treatment approaches.

In this part we share some of the most effective vestibular rehabilitation exercises, complete with instructions (with a warning that individuals should only do the exercises with the permission of their physician); suggestions on dietary changes, relaxation techniques, and herbal and nutritional supplements; and the benefits and pitfalls of surgical approaches.

I can honestly say that I don't have a burning desire to ride the world's fastest or highest roller coasters; and to those who do, good luck. What I do want is for people who suffer with dizziness, vertigo, or balance problems to find the help they need and deserve. Many of them don't realize that help is available, and that's why I wrote this book.

It is my hope that this book will guide you safely and easily through the dizzying process of discovery and understanding so you can find effective, satisfying treatment that allows you or your loved ones to live your lives to the fullest, without fear of falling, causing an accident, embarrassing yourself, or losing the level of activity you once enjoyed.

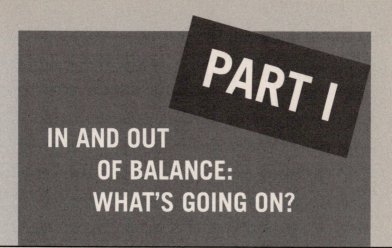

PART I

IN AND OUT OF BALANCE: WHAT'S GOING ON?

One minute you're walking down the street, feeling fine and confident, and then a split second later, a feeling of lightheadedness or dizziness overtakes you. It disappears quickly, or perhaps it doesn't, and you have to lean against a wall until the feeling passes while you wonder, "What's going on?"

Or as you get out of bed in the morning, the room begins to spin and you feel nauseous. Again, the symptoms may go away in a few seconds, or they may not, and you wait, frightened, for a few minutes or even longer until they do. Perhaps a similar episode happened to you weeks or even months ago, and you thought it was just a fluke. But now you're wondering, "What's going on?"

Or maybe you've been having some trouble with your balance lately, along with some lightheadedness and slight hearing loss. You're afraid to pick up your grandkids because you're fearful of losing your balance, so while you're watching the children play, you're wondering, "What's going on?"

It's a question tens of millions of Americans ask every year. It's a simple question, yet the answers are not always so. If you have a cold, take two aspirin, drink lots of fluids, and rest. If you're dizzy or experiencing a spinning feeling or losing your balance, what do you do? Hope it goes away? Live with the stress of wondering when the feeling will come again? If you want to go to a doctor, who should you see? Will you be able to accurately explain everything you've been experiencing? Do you know what information is important to tell your doctor?

In part I, we discuss the answers to these and other questions. You'll learn what you need to know about dizziness, vertigo, and balance problems so you can talk to your doctor and provide useful information that will help him or her arrive at an accurate diagnosis. You'll also learn how to find the right doctor to reach that diagnosis.

1

In Balance

If we were to ask you to name your senses, chances are you would list sight, smell, taste, hearing, and touch. These are the five basic senses our teachers told us about back in grade school. Few people, however, ever think to mention the "other" sense—balance, or equilibrium. Balance is a sense so many of us take for granted, that is, until something goes wrong and we "lose" it. That's when we discover that without our sense of balance, we find it virtually impossible to walk across a room, step up or off a curb, ride a bicycle, or get out of a chair or bed without crumbling into a heap onto the ground.

Most people have experienced one or more brief or fleeting episodes of losing their balance: feelings of dizziness, lightheadedness, or even vertigo (feeling as though either you or the world is spinning or whirling violently). You may experience a loss of balance if you rise too quickly from a bed or chair, have a serious bout of the flu or a head cold, drink too much alcohol, or ride a ferris wheel.

But millions of Americans experience feelings of being off-balance that are chronic or severe enough to make routine, every-day activities difficult. Chances are if you picked up this book, you or someone you love is among those millions. Perhaps you, like many of them, can no longer drive. Maybe you have trouble continuing to perform at your job, or maybe you can't find a job. You may be afraid to leave your house because you never know when you will become too dizzy or off-balance to maneuver across the street or to climb the stairs, go shopping, or even walk down to your mailbox.

As if the sensations of dizziness or being off-balance were not enough, you may often also experience other, associated symptoms that disrupt your life, such as nausea, vomiting, muscle aches in your neck and back, difficulty with concentration, headache, fatigue, muscle weakness, hearing loss, ringing in your ears (tinnitus), and increased sensitivity to light and noise.

As a result, your family and social lives suffer, and you may become angry, frightened, and depressed. You and millions of others like you get tired of going from doctor to doctor, looking for answers and finding none or unsatisfactory ones, answers that don't provide you with the relief you need and deserve. You feel as if your condition—whatever it is—has taken over your life.

If you or someone you care about suffers with dizziness or equilibrium problems, take heart. You are not alone, and there *is* help available.

This book offers you that help. In this chapter, we take the first steps with you and begin with a discussion of the components of your balance system and how it works—and what happens when it doesn't work—to keep you on your feet.

Accurate diagnosis of balance disorders is challenging for several reasons, not least of which are that dozens of factors can be involved and that many doctors are not well versed in the intricacies of the balance system. Therefore, you will find some technical information in the following pages. We encourage you to read through these pages, because they will help you understand the causes of balance problems.

As you will soon discover in the pages ahead, you—and other people who suffer with dizziness and other balance-related symptoms—play an integral role in the diagnosis and effective treatment of your disorder. You need to be able to accurately describe your experiences and related symptoms to your doctor, and such descriptions are not always easy unless you have the tools. One of the purposes of this book is to give you those tools. The more you understand the basics of how your balance system works, the better you will be able to tell your doctor about your symptoms and work with him or her to identify and find the most effective treatment approach for you.

Introducing Your Balance System

If you've always thought that your sense of balance is only in your head, think again. Balance is a complex system made up of three main components:

- The inner ear and neural (nerve) complex, which includes parts of the brain, specifically the brain stem and cerebellum. Altogether these elements are referred to as the *vestibular system*. This is a phrase we will use a lot in this book.
- The eyes, or visual system.
- The sensory system, also referred to as the proprioceptive system, which includes the skin, muscles, tendons, joints, and all their receptors which help you sense your environment. *Proprioceptive* is another term you will see a lot in the following chapters.

Thus, your sense of balance is really a whole-body experience—from your brain to your feet, and areas in between. And it is a learned experience: it takes a baby about two years to achieve a relatively stable sense of balance on two legs, and another year to be able to stand on one leg. Our sense of balance continues to perfect itself as we mature and as the brain and muscles become stronger and more coordinated.

If you suddenly feel off-balance or dizzy, it could be due to a faulty visual cue (say, you're having difficulty focusing with new glasses), a poor sensory cue (a loss of sensation in your foot when you take a step), an inner ear problem (an infection due to the flu or a more serious condition), or any combination of the three. In addition, another consideration is how the brain interprets the signals it receives from each of these areas.

The fact that balance is a sense that depends on many body parts and systems is important to keep in mind as you read this book. Balance—and the ability to maintain it—is a complex issue, and uncovering the reasons why you or a loved one may be experiencing dizziness, vertigo, or disequilibrium sometimes requires that doctors explore many different avenues. With that in mind, let's start at the beginning and explore the components of balance and their relationships with each other.

The Inner Ear

The inner ear is a very fragile environment that houses some very important organs of hearing and balance. Thus it is well protected and not readily accessible from the outside world. Here's what we mean.

JOURNEY TO THE INNER EAR

To get to the inner ear, you must first move past the outer ear, which consists of the *pinna* (flap made of cartilage) and the auditory canal, which is the tube that goes from the outer ear to the middle ear. Sound travels along this canal to reach the middle ear, an air-filled space less than 1 inch high and ¼ inch wide. The eardrum is stretched across the end of the auditory canal and is attached to three bones—the anvil, hammer, and stirrup—which together make up the *ossicles*. Sound waves travel across the ossicles, which cause them to vibrate, and the vibrations are then sent along to the inner ear (see Figures 1A and B).

INSIDE THE INNER EAR

The inner ear chamber is called the *labyrinth* (another word you'll see a lot of in this book). The labyrinth is encased in bone, and unlike the middle ear, the inner ear contains structures that are filled with liquids—*endolymph* and *perilymph*. These fluids bathe the nerve endings of the inner ear.

Two structures called the *oval window* and *round window* keep the liquid in and the air out of the inner ear. Beyond the windows lie the intricate structures and formations of the inner ear (see the figures to help you understand the relationship between these structures):

• *Cochlea.* This is a bony, coiled tube the size of a pea that is lined with cells with hairlike projections and filled with liquid. It is the organ of hearing, not balance. However, all the other structures in the inner ear—which are involved in balance—and the cochlea share a common blood supply; problems that affect the balance structures will also often affect the cochlea. This means that dizziness and balance problems are often accompanied by problems such as ringing in the ear and hearing difficulties.

• *Semicircular canals.* The semicircular canals are three fluid-filled tubes or loops (the anterior, posterior, and horizontal canals), each of which contains sensory cells called hair cells due to the appearance of hairlike structures on top of each cell. The canals are positioned at right angles to each other; this allows them to detect movement in any direction. Thus, one canal detects movements from side to side, another backward and forward, and the other up and down. In many cases, the hair cells in

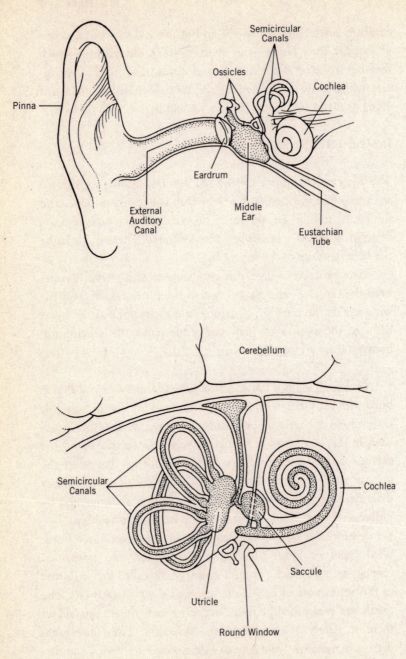

Figures 1A and B

all three of the canals are working simultaneously, bending as you move your head in various directions and sending signals to the brain via the *vestibular nerve.*

•   *Ampulla.* This is an enlarged area that appears at the end of each semicircular canal where it enters the vestibule. Each ampulla contains a *cupula,* a jellylike membrane that contains hair cells. When you move, the hair cells bend and send signals to the brain to let it know in which direction you are moving.

•   *Vestibule.* Each of the semicircular canals ends at an open area called the vestibule. This space contains two structures that are critical to balance: the *utricle* and *saccule,* which are sensitive to gravity. These gravitational sensors detect the position of the head and tell you whether you are upright in your environment. Inside the utricle and saccule is an otolithic membrane, a jellylike substance that is embedded with microscopic crystals called *otoconia.*

•   *Otoconia.* Also known as "ear stones" or "ear rocks," the otoconia are composed of calcium carbonate and protein. They respond to gravity by causing the hair cells in the sensory structures to bend in response to a change in the position of the head. These hair cells then send messages to the brain, via the vestibular nerve, where the signals are interpreted to determine your position, that is, if you're upright, off-balance, or upside down.

THE INNER EAR AT WORK

Collectively, the balance structures in the inner ear fall into two main categories: rotation sensors (the semicircular canals, ampulla, and cupula), which together help orient you when you turn your head in any direction; and gravity sensors (the utricle, saccule, and otoconia), which help you know which way is down. In an area the size of a dime, these tiny structures are always at work, constantly monitoring the position and movements of your head and sending signals to the brain for interpretation. Here are a few examples of how the inner ear works.

Say you're driving your car down the street toward a neighborhood playground, and you have your young daughter seated in the front seat next to you. Your eyes are on the road, when suddenly your daughter begins to cry. You quickly turn your head about 45 degrees to your right to see what the problem is. When you turn your head, several things happen. The fluid in the semicircular canals (called endolymph fluid) prompts the hairs to bend against the cells. The cells send nerve signals to the brain to rebalance your body as needed. At the same time, the signals are also telling your brain to turn your eyes 45 degrees to the left.

Of course, because you are a responsible driver and mother, you don't let your eyes linger too long on your child, as you may cause an accident, so you quickly return your head and eyes to a forward position. If you are healthy and your rotation sensors are operating properly, you can do this type of rapid sideways movement without feeling dizzy.

For example, when you turn your head to the right, the flow of endolymph fluid in the semicircular canals makes your eyes move to the left. That's when the balance mechanism that causes your eyes to turn to the left automatically adjusts them to match the same position as your head, thus avoiding dizziness or feeling off-balance.

Your gravity sensors also help you maintain your balance. You've arrived at your destination, and your daughter gets out of the car and begins to run toward the swings and slides. As she moves forward, the otoconia push back against the hairs in her utricle, acting as though she were falling backward. When her brain gets the information from the inner ear, it sends messages to the muscles, which rebalance her body and make it lean forward, thus restoring her balance. All of this happens in microseconds, so neither you nor she can detect that she could fall.

Similarly, say you're riding in the backseat of a car and you're seated behind the driver. The driver makes an unexpected turn to the left, which sends your body tilting or falling to the right. Immediately your gravity sensors tell your brain that you're tilting to the right, which then prompts a signal to the muscles in your leg or arm to push down against the seat or floor to counteract your fall toward the seat or the far door of the car.

Visual System

As you've probably already gathered by our discussion of the inner ear, your eyes supply your brain with a great deal of information that is processed for the purpose of helping you maintain your balance. At the most basic level is simple visual input. When light passes through the lens in your eyes and is focused on the retina, the images are recorded and transmitted by cells called cones and rods that connect to the optic nerve. The optic nerve then sends the messages to the areas of the brain responsible for vision.

At another level are two reflex systems that play a critical role in balance: the pursuit system, which is voluntary, and the optokinetic system, which is involuntary. The pursuit system allows your eyes to watch an object move across your field of vision without moving your head.

For example, you may stand in your front doorway and wave goodbye to your friends as they pull out of your driveway. Your eyes follow the movement of the car as it backs up, stops, and then shifts into forward motion. Up to a certain point, you don't need to move your head to see the movement of the car. Once the car travels outside the range your eyes can rotate, you will have to move your head to follow your friends' progress. The decision to move your head is voluntary.

The optokinetic system is an involuntary one in which your eyes move when your field of view moves. For example, have you ever looked out the window of a plane as it is backing away from the terminal and felt as if the area outside the plane—and not you—was moving? Your eyes were sending a message to the brain that your environment was moving, but other parts of your balance system—like your sense of touch or the semicircular canals in your inner ear—were sending signals that *you* were moving. Some people are not bothered by the conflicting messages, but others are and they can feel dizzy or off-balance, if only for a few seconds.

Sometimes we intentionally send mixed messages to the brain. Remember playing pin the tail on the donkey? In that game, people are blindfolded, spun around, and then told to pin a paper tail on a picture of a donkey hanging on a wall. Here's what happens when you play this game.

One, spinning temporarily disturbs the movement of fluid in your inner ear. When you spin, the fluid stimulates the hair cells in the canals, which in turn activate a signal from the vestibular nerve to the brain. When you stop spinning, the fluid still moves for a few seconds, so your brain keeps receiving the message that you are still moving, and so you feel dizzy. This is a normal—and temporary—response. But in a matter of seconds, or perhaps up to a minute, the dizziness disappears.

Two, you have been deprived of your vision, so you cannot use visual information to help you determine your body's position in relation to your surroundings. The combination of these two factors—spinning and having no visual cues—can make you lose your balance or feel dizzy for longer than if you had not been blindfolded.

Here's yet one more example of how your visual system is involved in dizziness and balance. Can you read while traveling in a car, train, or bus without feeling nauseous? Many people can't, and here's why. When you are moving, your inner ears are sending information to your brain synchronous with your movement. Your eyes, however, are fixed on your reading material and fail to reveal to your brain the same visual conditions it expects to see as they relate to the inner ear information. Such conflicting information causes the nausea and dizziness we refer to as motion sickness.

Sensory System

The sensory, or proprioceptive, system includes the muscles, tendons, skin, and joints throughout the body. The signals from these structures, such as pressure against the bottom of your feet as you stand, the twist of your ankle as you step off a curb, or the touch of the bannister under your hand as you climb stairs, travel from your hands and feet and other sites to the brain. Your muscles are constantly contracting and relaxing, in response to the surfaces you come into contact with as well as the Earth's gravitational pull. The messages they send to the brain come from sensory receptors called *proprioceptors,* and the information they send is known as *proprioceptive input.*

Although all the signals sent to your brain via the proprioceptors are helpful in maintaining equilibrium, those which come from the neck (which signals which way your head is moving) and ankles (which signal the position of your body in relation to the surface beneath your feet) are the most important. Your brain interprets this information, along with the signals it receives from your eyes and inner ear, to help you maintain your proper positioning.

Bringing It All Together: The Brain

The brain is the central relay station for all the signals that are transmitted to it from your inner ear, eyes, muscles, joints, tendons, and skin. Two areas of the brain that are most responsible for balance are the brain stem, which helps maintain posture, and the cerebellum, which is located just above the brain stem and controls your muscles.

When all systems are go—when the brain and the other three systems are healthy and functioning properly—the brain receives symmetrical (balanced), accurate, and consistent information. Once the messages reach the brain, they are interpreted by the brain, which then sends out signals to the extraocular (eye) muscles and to the muscles in the body. These signals allow for adjustments in eye position that help keep your eyes in synch with your surroundings. They also allow your muscles to make the necessary modifications to correctly place your body in relation to your environment and maintain balance.

BRAIN COMPENSATION

Usually the brain can compensate when it receives inadequate, mixed, or no sensory information. For example, what if you are staying overnight in an unfamiliar room and you get up in the middle of the night to go to the bathroom. You forget where the light switch is, so in the pitch darkness, you need to depend on your sense of touch (perhaps by running your hand along the wall and carefully stepping with your feet) to guide you until you reach a light. In such a situation, even without visual cues, your brain will receive enough information from your sense of touch to help you stay balanced.

The brain also compensates after the vestibular sensors in the inner ear are damaged or injured. Even if one of your inner ears was completely destroyed, your brain would compensate: it would utilize the input from your remaining healthy inner ear better and make adjustments so that your balance system would function.

Thus when signals are confusing or inadequate (e.g., your ears are plugged because of a cold, your eyes are closed, or you are walking on a soft surface like a sandy beach), your brain can compensate by using information it receives from other areas to determine your body's position and maintain your balance. Like breathing, all of the messages sent to the brain and the adjustments the brain makes are done automatically, without conscious thought, and we go about our lives expecting them to remain so.

But sometimes, something goes wrong. What if your brain can't compensate? What if you have a disease or injury and there is little or no information reaching the brain?

Going Out of Balance

As we already discussed, if you put on a blindfold and spin around, you're likely to get dizzy, at least for a few seconds. The lack of visual input from your eyes, along with the fact that the fluid in your inner ears stays in motion for a few seconds after you physically stop moving, results in dizziness. Indeed, most people can expect to feel dizzy or off-balance temporarily if they intentionally spin around or take a ride on a roller coaster.

Let's return to that dark, unfamiliar room in the middle of the night. What if you had arthritis, a stroke, Parkinson's disease, multiple sclerosis, diabetes, or another health condition that compromised your sense of touch and pressure. The signals transmitted to your brain from your muscles and skin could be interrupted or misinterpreted, your reflexes could be slowed or compromised, and you could lose your balance.

Many people also experience damage to their inner ear. Sometimes, depending on the extent of the injury, the brain takes longer to compensate for damage that has occurred to various parts of the balance system. The result can be weeks, months, even years of living with dizziness and balance problems. This can happen to people of any age but especially to older individuals, as you'll read about in chapter 8 and other sections of this book. Fortunately, in many cases there is an excellent way you can help your brain compensate, and actually speed up the healing process. That method is called vestibular rehabilitation therapy, which we discuss in detail in chapter 12.

Bottom Line

Maintaining your balance requires the cooperation and synchronization of signals from your vestibular, visual, and proprioceptive systems, which are orchestrated by the brain. When all parts of all these systems are in harmony, you probably don't give your sense of balance a second thought.

But there are dozens of factors that can affect these three systems and ultimately impact your equilibrium. For many people, feelings of dizziness, disequilibrium, or vertigo are the result of something that goes wrong in the inner ear, visual system, proprioceptive system, or brain. Perhaps they have an infection in or injury to the inner ear. They may have a visual problem in one or both eyes that causes their inner ear and eyes to be out of synch. They may have a medical condition, such as multiple sclerosis, arthritis, diabetes, circulation problems, or a head injury, that causes weakened or disturbed signals to be sent to the brain.

The rest of this book focuses on those times when something goes wrong—from minor, temporary episodes of dizziness to serious, debilitating cases of vertigo and disequilibrium—what conditions exist at those times, and what you can do about them. First we'll turn to the basics: the three types of balance disorders and how to identify them.

2

Off-balance: I'm So Dizzy

In this chapter, we're going to help you accurately describe the sensations you are experiencing when you say "I'm dizzy" or "I feel off-balance" or "I had an attack of vertigo." We will explore different types of dizziness, vertigo, and disequilibrium and how to distinguish between them. When you're through with this chapter, you'll be equipped to explain how you feel to your doctor.

You may be wondering why we're dedicating an entire chapter to explanations of these three types of balance disorders. Because these three words—"Doctor, I'm dizzy"—uttered by approximately 50 percent of the people in the United States at least once during their lives, can cause many a physician's heart to skip a beat. That's because dizzy patients are among the most difficult patients to treat. We don't say this to discourage you, but as a way to preface our discussion of what it means to be dizzy or off-balance or to experience vertigo, because these feelings are hard to describe in words. Ten different people can go to their doctors complaining of feeling dizzy, and each of them may have a different way of explaining how they feel.

Difficult does not mean impossible. But in order for your health-care practitioners to correctly diagnose these conditions and then choose the best treatment approach, it's necessary for you to:

- Understand the difference between dizziness, vertigo, and disequilibrium. They are *not* the same, and in this chapter we'll show you how they are different.
- Explain your symptoms to your doctor using words that most accurately describe what you experience. We have included a detailed dizziness questionnaire for you to complete and bring with you to your doctor's office.
- Realize that it's possible for you to experience dizziness, vertigo, *and* disequilibrium. Then again, of the three symptoms, you may experience dizziness only. As we said earlier, diagnosing dizzy patients is not an easy task.

Let's take the first steps in eliminating dizziness, vertigo, and/or disequilibrium from your life—understanding the culprits. Because providing accurate information to your health-care practitioners is so important, we suggest you begin by keeping a journal.

Your Dizzy Journal

Your dizzy journal can be any type of notebook, diary, or other convenient way to record your thoughts and specific experiences surrounding any episodes of dizziness, vertigo, and/or problems with balance. Most people prefer to keep a written record, although some find it more convenient to use a handheld tape recorder to document their thoughts. The important thing is to record *anything* that may be helpful to your doctor.

As you read about each of the three types of balance disorders in this chapter, we will tell you which elements to look for and note in your journal. Do not, however, feel that you are limited to these suggestions. If you experience other symptoms you believe may be relevant or there are situations in your life that you believe may have an impact on how you're feeling, please note them as well. It's better to have too much information than not enough.

Vertigo

Many people have the misconception that vertigo is merely a case of severe dizziness, but in fact these two conditions are different (see "Dizziness" later in this chapter). If you understand the difference and can explain your sensations accurately to your doctor, then he or she will have a better idea of how to approach your care.

Vertigo is the illusion that either you or the environment around you is spinning, rotating, rolling, rocking, or whirling. In some cases, people experience the sensation of tilting. If you're riding a carousel, you expect to feel as though you are spinning, and in fact, you are. But if you feel as though you are turning while standing in your living room or office or if you feel as though the world around you is whirling when you try to get out of bed in the morning, then you're experiencing an episode of vertigo.

The sensations of vertigo can last for seconds, minutes, hours, or even days or months, and they can be mild to severe. They may happen just once during your lifetime, they may happen more than once but infrequently, or they may happen often.

If you experience prolonged, debilitating, or increasingly worse episodes of vertigo, you should see your doctor immediately, especially if vision difficulties, problems with swallowing or speaking, headache, weakness in your legs or arms, or mental confusion accompany your vertigo.

CAUSES OF VERTIGO

Vertigo is not a disease in itself but a symptom, an indication that there's been some kind of damage, abuse, or other factor that has adversely affected the vestibular system. There are dozens of situations that can cause or contribute to vertigo attacks, including but not limited to viral infections, allergies, ear diseases, trauma to the head or ear, and neurological disorders. These and other conditions are discussed in part II of this book, "Why Am I So Dizzy? Causes of Balance Disorders."

UNCOVERING THE ELEMENTS OF VERTIGO

In chapters 3 and 10, we talk about the general and specific tests, respectively, your doctor may conduct to uncover why you are experiencing vertigo. You can help your doctor better diagnose and ultimately treat your condition by providing him or her with all the details of your vertigo episodes. Here are the elements which you should consider and about which your doctor will question you. Your journal is a good place to keep an accurate record of these elements.

Time Element. The duration of your vertigo episodes can provide a clue as to whether there is a specific disease involved or another reason for the sensations. Episodes that last seconds, for example, indicate benign paroxysmal positional vertigo. Those that last minutes suggest different disorders from episodes that span hours.

Accompanying Symptoms. Often, vertigo is accompanied by other symptoms. These associated symptoms can also provide clues and help doctors identify the cause of your condition. Symptoms you may experience include sweating, paleness, nausea, vomiting, ringing in the ears, a sensation of pressure in the inner ear, hearing loss, and problems with balance and coordination. Note these and any other symptoms in your journal.

Some attacks of vertigo are accompanied by nystagmus, a series of involuntary eye movements, usually side to side. (We discuss nystagmus again in chapter 3.) The movement of the pupil to one side is slower than the movement to the other side, which results in a jerking motion in one direction.

After the sensation of spinning or whirling has disappeared, many people report feeling out of balance or unsteady for a while. These feelings are common, as the brain needs to compensate for the vertigo episode. Generally, recovery time from an attack takes a little longer in older individuals because the brain needs more time to adjust. You should always make a note of the time it takes for you to recover so you can tell your doctor.

Precipitating Factors. "All I did was turn over in bed, and suddenly the entire room was spinning," says Brenda, a 43-year-old sales representative. What Brenda experienced was vertigo that occurs as the result of a sudden change in position, such as sitting up suddenly from a prone position, bending over and straightening up, or looking up. This is commonly referred to as positional vertigo.

Changes in middle ear pressure, which can occur when you cough, sneeze, or fly in a plane, can also bring on an attack of vertigo, as can a sudden loud noise, which may damage the inner ear. Keep in mind that the event that triggers your episode of vertigo may not always be obvious, so it is best to tell your doctor about any situation or event that immediately preceded your vertigo attack. Even if you don't believe something is important, it may be more relevant than you think it is.

Dizziness

The term *dizziness* is a very general one, so experts created categories to help doctors better diagnose and manage patients. The first thing you need to do is understand that there is a difference between *dizziness* and *vertigo*. In simplest terms, vertigo is a form of dizziness characterized by the sensation that either you or your environment is whirling or spinning; feelings of lightheadedness, faintness, or giddiness are termed *dizziness*.

You can assist your doctor in making a diagnosis if you better understand what dizziness is and better explain your sensations to your doctor. To help you reach that understanding, let's look at some common types of dizziness.

Here's a helpful hint: If all this talk about dizziness and vertigo is *making* you dizzy, relax. Our goal is to eliminate, not cause, dizziness. Simply note your feelings and sensations in your journal without using the words *dizzy* or *vertigo*. The following explanations of the different types of dizziness will help you do just that.

NEAR-FAINT DIZZINESS

If you've ever risen up suddenly from a seated or lying position or stood up quickly after you've been squatting down gardening for a while, you may have experienced a brief sensation of lightheadedness. You may even have felt as if you might fall or faint; perhaps you had to reach out to hold onto a wall or chair.

What you experienced is commonly called near-faint dizziness or presyncope (as compared with syncope, which is a full faint, or complete loss of consciousness). Many people believe that near-faint dizziness is a symptom of an impending stroke, but this is not the case. In fact, in the majority of cases, this type of dizziness is nothing more than a minor inconvenience. In some people, however, it does indicate a more serious problem. Different causes of near-faint dizziness, such as orthostatic hypotension, hyperventilation, and heart problems, are discussed in part II.

PSYCHOPHYSIOLOGIC DIZZINESS

A clear example of the power of mind over matter and the mind-body connection is the occurrence of dizziness related to psychiatric conditions. The fact that the mind is the source of the dizziness doesn't make the sensation any less disturbing or real, however.

Psychophysiologic dizziness may occur periodically or constantly, and last for months or years. Sensations of lightheadedness, dissociation (feeling as if you've left your body), giddiness, or floating are typically accompanied by other symptoms, including but not limited to shortness of breath, heart palpitations, sweating, nausea, urinary problems, backache, general weakness, and fatigue.

Dizziness and its accompanying symptoms usually begin after a stressful event, such as the death of a loved one, divorce, or a serious illness, or when faced with a situation that causes panic, such as having to drive over a bridge or get into an elevator. Dizziness that is driven by psychological conditions is discussed in chapter 9.

OCULAR DIZZINESS

Ocular dizziness is a type of dizziness associated with eye problems, such as cataracts or glaucoma, or use of visual aids, such as glasses or contact lenses. Oscillopsia, a condition in which people believe that stationary objects are moving up and down or back and forth, is much less common but is another type of ocular dizziness. Chapter 8 discusses the different conditions that can cause or contribute to ocular dizziness.

MULTISENSORY DIZZINESS

The term *multisensory dizziness* is used to describe dizziness that involves several senses, such as a diminished sense of touch and pressure, a weakened vestibular system, and poor vision. This type of dizziness is most common in elderly individuals and in those who have diabetes, multiple sclerosis, or other medical conditions that involve a reduction in sensory perception. Chapter 8 looks at some of these disorders.

PHYSIOLOGIC DIZZINESS

Physiologic dizziness occurs in healthy individuals whose visual, vestibular, or proprioceptive systems are physically stimulated in a way that creates mismatched signals. For example, riding in the backseat of a car causes some people to get motion sickness, which results when what they see isn't in synch with the signals being sent by their inner ear. Height sickness is another type of physiologic dizziness. Physiologic dizziness is related to the inner ear and is discussed in chapters 4 and 5.

DRUG-INDUCED DIZZINESS

When you get home from the doctor's office or pharmacy with a new prescription, the last thing you want to deal with is side effects from the very medications you've been given to (hopefully) make you feel better. Yet the number of prescription and nonprescription drugs that can cause dizziness is itself staggering: dizziness is a side effect of approximately 25 percent of the drugs listed in the *Physician's Desk Reference* (a standard drug reference book; see Suggested Reading). Another type of drug that is often associated with dizziness is alcohol.

Medications that cause dizziness and other adverse effects on balance and hearing are called ototoxic drugs. Episodes of dizziness related to ototoxic medication use are divided into two categories: reversible and irreversible. In chapter 9, we discuss both types of otoxicity, as well as those drugs that are more likely to cause vertigo or disequilibrium.

Disequilibrium

Many people say they are dizzy when in fact what they are experiencing is disequilibrium—imbalance or unsteadiness. The sensation of being unsteady, or in a state of disequilibrium, occurs only when people are standing or walking, not when they are sitting or lying down. Disequilibrium may or may not be accompanied by dizziness or vertigo.

To better understand disequilibrium, it helps to understand what equilibrium is. Equilibrium is correlated to *postural control,* which involves the ability to maintain the vertical alignment of the body and its parts to counteract the forces of gravity and to remain upright. Thus disequilibrium is the inability to maintain control of your posture and to remain on your feet.

Although imbalance can affect people of any age, it is especially common among older people because they are more likely to have deficits in their vestibular, visual, and proprioceptive systems. One major concern about disequilibrium among older people is the risk of falling and suffering a fracture (see "Aging" below).

CAUSES OF DISEQUILIBRIUM

Like vertigo and dizziness, disequilibrium is a symptom and not a disease. It also can have many different causes, including but not limited to aging, tumors, chronic diseases, poor circulation, infections of the inner ear, and psychological conditions. These and other causes of disequilibrium are covered in part II.

UNCOVERING THE ELEMENTS OF DISEQUILIBRIUM

Feelings of imbalance and unsteadiness differ from person to person, and how they manifest depends on their source. Therefore the better you can describe the sensations and associated symptoms you experience with your imbalance, the better your doctor can diagnose and treat your condition.

A Matter of Degree. Your doctor will want to know the degree of your sensations. Do you have a vague feeling of imbalance, one that doesn't knock you off your feet but leaves you feeling generally unsteady? Do you feel unsteady most or all of the time, so much so that the feeling disrupts your life? Is your sense of balance worse when you are in the dark or in poorly lit surroundings? Your answer to these questions will help your health-care practitioner zero in on your condition.

Accompanying Symptoms. Disequilibrium does not occur in a vacuum; other symptoms accompany it, symptoms that can offer your doctor crucial clues as to the cause of your balance problem. Symptoms that are often seen along with disequilibrium include acute vertigo, hearing loss, oscillopsia (an illusion that inanimate or stationary objects are moving up and down or left and right), loss of coordination, muscle weakness or numbness in the extremities, bowel and bladder dysfunction, and slowed movements. Generally, report any symptom that immediately preceded the disequilibrium or occurred since you first noticed the disequilibrium.

Aging. One of the natural changes that occurs with the aging process is a change in gait, which affects balance. Older women tend to have a slight waddle to their walk, while older men tend to take shorter steps and swing their arms less. For many older people, these changes don't significantly affect their ability to walk or do their regular daily activities.

In some people, however, especially as they reach their eighties, their gait is eventually reduced to a shuffle. They have difficulty making a turn or pivot, and when getting up from a seated position, they find it difficult to take the first step. Naturally, balance is a problem for these individuals, and with it comes a great fear of falling. The risk of falling increases after age 60, and women are more susceptible to falls than men. Unfortunately, older women are also at higher risk of osteoporosis, and so a fall for them too often means a fracture as well. That's one reason why uncovering the cause of disequilibrium and treating it promptly is important.

Another problem associated with aging and disequilibrium is the use of medications. Older people are more likely than younger ones to be taking several over-the-counter and prescription drugs at the same time, and any one or more of them may be contributing to or causing their balance problems. Make sure you tell your health-care practitioner about all medications you are taking, as well as any vitamins or herbal remedies.

The Dizziness Questionnaire

The information I gather about the history of my patients' dizziness is, in my opinion, more important than the physical signs of their balance disorder. Accurate information about the time of onset of the complaint, any precipitating events (e.g., when symptoms first occurred—while driving, during or immediately after an illness, or while flying), the frequency of the symptoms, and any associated symptoms are valuable clues to the root of the problem.

First it is necessary to identify the chief complaint, as we've already discussed; that is, are you experiencing dizziness, vertigo, or disequilibrium? The best way to accurately identify the complaint is for you to complete a dizziness questionnaire. The dizziness questionnaire does not take the place of a complete medical history. Rather, it focuses on factors that are especially relevant to balance disorders, and the information gathered is evaluated along with the medical history data.

Not all physicians use the same questionnaire. Some physicians have incorporated a dizziness questionnaire into their medical history forms; others have a separate form for you to complete. The sample questions presented in the box are an example of the type of information your doctors may request. You can prepare for your doctor's visit by answering these questions at home and bringing the answers with you, along with any notes you've made in your journal. Both the questionnaire and your journal are valuable tools in uncovering the cause of your dizziness or balance problems, and as an extension, in finding the most appropriate treatment.

DIZZINESS QUESTIONNAIRE

PRIMARY SYMPTOMS

Which of the following phrases accurately describe your dizziness? Mark all that apply.

- Lightheaded
- Giddy
- Feeling like I'm going to fall
- Feeling like objects around me are spinning or turning
- Feeling like I'm spinning or turning but objects around me are not
- Tilting or leaning
- Swimming sensation in my head
- Headache
- Nausea
- Vomiting
- Tendency to veer to the left when walking in the dark
- Tendency to veer to the right when walking in the dark
- Feeling of pressure in my head
- Feeling of pressure in my ear(s)
- Tingling in my hands or toes or around my mouth
- Loss of consciousness

TIME OF ONSET AND CONTRIBUTING FACTORS

- When did you first experience feelings of dizziness?

- How often do you have dizzy spells?
- How long do the spells last?
- How do you feel in between your dizzy spells?
- Do the dizzy spells occur at a particular time of day?
- Do any of the following make your dizziness worse or trigger it?
  - Hunger
  - Menstrual period
  - Bending your head forward or backward
  - Turning your head to either side
  - Coughing
  - Bowel movement
  - Stress
  - Fatigue
  - Drinking alcohol
  - Flying
  - Driving or riding in a moving vehicle
  - Heights (e.g., looking down from a balcony or a window in a high-rise building)
  - Ingesting caffeine (including coffee, tea, colas, chocolate)
  - Using tobacco
  - Using any particular medication (over-the-counter and prescription)

ASSOCIATED SYMPTOMS

Indicate whether you also experience any of the following symptoms. Mark all that apply.

- Difficulty hearing (If yes, which ear)
- Ringing in the ear(s) (If yes, which ear)
- Pressure or stuffiness in the ear(s)
- Pain in the ear(s)
- Discharge from the ear(s)

- Blurred vision
- Double vision
- Numbness in the face or extremities
- Loss of consciousness
- Difficulty swallowing

RELEVANT MEDICAL HISTORY

- Do you have any allergies? (Describe; include airborne, food, drug, etc.)
- Have you ever had a head injury? (Explain; include at what age(s) and severity.)
- Did you have earaches or ear infections as a child?
- Did you suffer with motion sickness before the age of 12 years?
- Have you experienced motion sickness within the last 10 years?
- Do you now have diabetes? High blood pressure? Kidney disease? Thyroid disease? Bouts of migraine? Heart disease?
- Do you have a family history of diabetes? Ear disease? Neurological disease (e.g., multiple sclerosis or Parkinson's disease)? Migraine?
- Are you taking any medications? (List them; include non-prescription and prescription.)
- Have you ever taken any medications for dizziness? (List them.)

Bottom Line

You can play a major role in the diagnosis and treatment of your balance disorder if you better understand your symptoms and what you need to tell your doctor about them. The next time you experience an episode of dizziness or imbalance, make notes in your journal:

- What preceded or precipitated the event? If you're not sure, write down what you think it might be.
- Describe how you felt, without using the words *dizzy, vertigo,* or *off-balance.*

An accurate description can be invaluable in uncovering the cause of your balance disorder. That being said, we're ready to go on to the next chapter, in which we talk about how you can find the right health-care practitioner(s) to help you, and the initial steps in the diagnostic process.

3

Getting a Diagnosis:
The First Steps

Now that you've learned about the differences between vertigo, disequilibrium, and various types of dizziness, you're better prepared to lend your doctor a hand in evaluating your condition and, ultimately, in deciding on a plan of action. But how does your doctor go about conducting that evaluation? We thought you'd ask that question.

Uncovering the reason why you are experiencing dizziness or a loss of balance requires two things: a doctor who is part detective, and a darn good one at that, and input from you. While the cause of some cases of dizziness are easy to identify—for example, you just started to take a new medication, they've just repainted your office at work, or you're suffering with a severe bout of the flu—others are much less obvious and require detective work. That may mean your physicians will need to thoroughly examine all three elements of your balance system—your vestibular system, eyes, and sense of touch and vibration—and then evaluate the information to arrive at a diagnosis and relevant treatment plan.

But the total burden of diagnosis is not on your health-care providers. The more information you can supply your doctors, the better they will be able to identify your condition. The more you understand why your doctors ask you certain questions and how the investigative process will go, the better they will be able to help you. A reciprocal, trusting relationship with your doctors is a critical part of successful health care.

That's why in this chapter we explain some of the various procedures and tests your health-care practitioners may perform during the initial diagnostic process. We say *initial* because if your primary care physician feels it is necessary to refer you to a specialist after he or she has completed your examination, you will then go on to a second phase of diagnosis, which we cover in chapter 11. In this chapter, we discuss the importance of completing a dizziness questionnaire and a comprehensive medical history, the components of the physical examination and why each one is done, and the neurological examination and what the different tests indicate.

Before you undergo any of these procedures, you need to choose a doctor. So we begin with *your* detective work by looking at the different types of doctors you may go to for help.

How to Find a Qualified Health-Care Practitioner

Balance problems and dizziness can affect many organs in the body; this means several medical specialists may be needed to diagnose and manage your condition. If you are like most people, the place to begin is with your primary care physician or internist. A primary care physician is usually the doctor patients see first with their complaints, and then they are referred to specialists as needed. Most primary physicians are internists, physicians who are trained in the diagnosis and nonsurgical treatment of disorders and diseases that affect the internal organs, such as cancer, infections, and diseases of the blood, heart, joints, kidneys, stomach, intestines, lungs, and reproductive organs. They also have an understanding of common conditions that affect the ears, eyes, skin, and nervous system.

Your primary care doctor will conduct a basic evaluation, which should include a medical history, a physical examination, and the completion of a detailed dizziness questionnaire. If you take this approach, hopefully your doctor will uncover a minor problem that can be resolved quickly or that, given a little time, will resolve itself. Typically, minor causes of dizziness can include:

- Cold or flu
- Fatigue
- Insomnia
- Sinus conditions, such as sinusitis
- Excessive stress
- Dehydration
- Fasting
- Extreme environmental temperature changes
- Heavy menstrual bleeding
- Adverse reaction to a medication, prescription or over-the-counter
- Ear infection

Naturally, some of these conditions may be associated with more serious conditions, but in most cases they can be remedied easily or will simply resolve themselves within a short time.

If the information your doctor has gathered doesn't lead to a definite diagnosis, he or she may conduct some tests that focus on the systems that he or she suspects may be involved. Some of those tests, including a magnetic resonance imaging (MRI) test to scan the brain, ultrasound of the arteries to see if you have any circulation problems, and blood tests to rule out anemia, are discussed below.

If your situation requires more detective work, your doctor will refer you to a specialist on the basis of the results of your basic evaluation. For example, if you are experiencing frequent or chronic bouts of low blood pressure or you have underlying heart disease, you will likely be referred to a cardiologist. If you are experiencing ringing in your ears or you feel as if the world is spinning around you, you'll be referred to an otorhinolaryngologist or neurotologist. If you are experiencing muscle weakness or severe headache, a neurologist may be in order.

It's important that you communicate your symptoms as accurately as possible to your primary care physician. The information you provide, along with the results of your examination and your medical history, can help your doctor either reach a diagnosis or decide which specialist you need to see.

You may, however, be among a smaller group of people who are already seeing a specialist for a medical condition, such as heart disease or diabetes. If you know or suspect your dizziness or balance symptoms are associated with a previously diagnosed medical problem, you may choose to bypass your primary care doctor and schedule an appointment with your specialist.

Several specialists are typically associated with the diagnosis and treatment of dizziness and balance disorders. Among them are cardiologists, endocrinologists, neurologists, neurotologists, orthopedic surgeons, otorhinolaryngologists (also called ear-nose-throat doctors, [ENTs]), neurosurgeons, and vascular surgeons. (Physical therapists, who are involved in evaluation and treatment regarding rehabilitation, are discussed in chapter 12.)

MEDICAL SPECIALTIES

Because most cases of dizziness or balance disorders involve the inner ear, the specialists people are most often referred to are otorhinolaryngologists or neurotologists. In some cases, one or more other medical specialists are called in to be part of the treatment team. Here's a brief description of the specialists to whom you may be referred.

• Neurotologists focus on ear and balance disorders. Neurotology is a subspecialty of otorhinolaryngology. Individuals in this subspecialty complete one to two years of training beyond the five years of otorhinolaryngology training.

• Otorhinolaryngologists, or ENTs, focus on the diagnosis and management of disorders and diseases of the ear, nose, throat, and related structures of the head and neck. After four years of medical school, individuals who choose this specialty pursue at least five additional years of training.

• Cardiologists focus on the prevention, diagnosis, and treatment of heart disease and other conditions that affect the heart, blood vessels, and lungs. Disorders that affect these structures can affect your sense of balance.

• Endocrinologists are internists who have chosen to subspecialize in disorders of the endocrine glands. These practitioners deal with disorders such as diabetes, pituitary diseases, and metabolic and nutritional ailments, all of which can play a role in dizziness and balance.

• Neurologists specialize in diseases and disorders of the brain and central nervous system, including those areas which control balance. Some of the conditions neurologists diagnose and treat include dementia, epilepsy, headache and migraine, multiple sclerosis, Parkinson's disease, and stroke. They complete at least three years of specialty training in neurology after medical school, and they can further their education still more by pursuing a one- or two-year fellowship studying one of these diseases or disorders.

• Neurosurgeons diagnose, evaluate, and treat disorders of the central, peripheral, and autonomic nervous systems. They are consulted when surgery may be indicated for disorders of the brain, meninges (membrane covering of the brain), pituitary gland, spinal cord, and spine. Tumors in any of these structures, as well as nerve problems that compromise the sense of touch, can play a role in dizziness and balance problems.

• Orthopedic surgeons specialize in the diagnosis and the medical and surgical treatment of diseases that affect the muscles, joints, and bones. Conditions may include injuries or infections associated with any of these structures, as well as diseases, such as osteoporosis, rheumatoid arthritis, and osteoarthritis.

• Vascular surgeons specialize in the surgical correction of conditions that affect the blood vessels.

Naturally, you won't need the services of all these medical professionals, and most people work with only one or two of them. But these experts may be among the most important people in your life if you are suffering with a chronic or debilitating balance problem.

HOW TO CHOOSE YOUR DOCTOR

To help you choose the most-experienced and compatible practitioners for your management team, consider the following guidelines when making your selections. If you are part of a health insurance plan that allows you to choose all of your own doctors, so much the better. If your plan limits your choice or doesn't give you one, it is still a good idea to know all you can about the doctor in whose hands you are placing your health.

• Where did the doctor attend medical school? The American Medical Association's Physician Select can verify your doctor's training and certification status. The service is free and can be accessed at www.ama-assn.org/aps/amahg.htm.

• Is the doctor board certified? To be board certified, doctors must meet high standards. The American Board of Medical Specialties Certified Doctor Verification Service can tell you if a doctor is certified in a specific field. This is a free service and can be found at www.abms.org/nwsearch.asp.

• Has the doctor ever been reprimanded by the state disciplinary board, been convicted of fraud, or had any action taken against him or her? You can check the state medical board in your state for a list of names of disciplined doctors. Many state medical boards include this information on their websites as well. A central location with links to the states' medical boards is the Public Citizen Research Group, which is at www.citizen.org/hrg/publications/1506.htm. The service is free.

• How many years has the doctor been practicing?

• Does the doctor have a solo or group practice? If your doctor is not available, will another doctor in the group see you instead?

• What health insurance does the doctor accept?

• Is the doctor or an associate available on weekends or at night?

• With which hospital or clinic is the doctor associated? Is this facility convenient for you? Is the facility one that is covered by your insurance plan?

• Are the doctor's office location and hours convenient for you?

• Is the doctor's staff friendly and helpful?

The Physical Examination

Not every doctor performs a physical examination in exactly the same way or to the same extent. Your doctor will choose the procedures and tests he or she believes are best for your situation. The following examination procedures are typical of those done by primary care physicians. If you are later referred to a specialist, he or she may repeat some of these examinations. A discussion of the various tests specialists may perform is found in chapter 11, "What to Expect If You Need Special Tests." Remember to bring your completed dizziness questionnaire and any notes with you to your examination. These will help your doctor with a diagnosis.

HEAD AND NECK EXAMINATION

The physical examination often begins with an evaluation of the head and neck. This is important because frequently, people who complain of dizziness have an ailment or condition that is affecting their ears, nose, eyes, head, or throat. Your doctor will use a stethoscope to listen for any abnormal sounds in your neck as the blood is pumped through the carotid artery (located on the side of the neck) to your brain. A disturbance in blood flow can affect balance and cause dizziness.

He or she will also look into your mouth to check the structures in your throat and mouth. Any abnormality, such as a tumor or other growth, can influence balance.

EAR EXAMINATION

When it comes to exploring your ears, a physical examination can only allow the doctor to see as far as the middle ear. The otoscope, the lighted, magnifying instrument doctors use to examine the ears, cannot see into the inner ear, where the balance system is located. An otoscope can, however, check for signs of an ear infection, ear wax buildup, trauma to the middle ear, or injury to the ear drum, all of which may play a role in dizziness. An otorhinolaryngologist or neurotologist can conduct the necessary tests for the inner ear (see chapter 11).

Although your internist can't see into your inner ear, he or she can do a simple test to determine if there is a hole, or fistula, in your inner ear. While you look straight ahead, the doctor will press on your ear with his or her hand. If your eyes spontaneously turn to one side or if you experience vertigo or dizziness, these signs may indicate an inner ear problem that needs further investigation by a specialist.

If you have been experiencing some hearing loss or distortion, your doctor may also conduct a simple hearing test. This is done using a vibrating tuning fork that the doctor will hold against your forehead or behind your ear. This test does not take the place of an audiogram, which is a sophisticated hearing test conducted in a soundproof room (see chapter 11). It can, however, signal that something may be amiss and prompt further examination by a specialist.

NEUROLOGICAL EXAMINATION

Your doctor may also conduct a brief neurological examination that includes some or all of the following tests. Your doctor will choose the tests that most appropriately match your symptoms: some of these tests can reveal information about a malfunction in the vestibular system, while others provide clues about your brain or sensory functioning.

• Reflex test. Your practitioner lightly taps your ankle and knee with a rubber-headed hammer to evaluate your nerve functioning.

• Muscle tone and strength test. To test muscle tone, your practitioner may move your legs or arms to see if there is a difference between the two sides of your body. A test of muscle strength usually involves you pushing against your doctor's hand or arm or squeezing his fingers.

• Coordination tests. How you perform such tasks as closing your eyes and placing your extended index finger on your nose, or flipping your hand palm side up and then palm side down on your thigh several times rapidly can indicate whether there is a malfunction in the cerebellum.

• Positional tests. To try to induce vertigo and nystagmus, the doctor will place you in various positions and note how your eyes respond. These tests are typically done as part of a battery of tests called electronystagmography, which is discussed in detail in chapter 11 (see "Electronystagmography Testing" in that chapter).

• Gait and posture tests. In addition to observing how you walk across the room, your doctor may conduct the following tests:

• In the Romberg test, you'll be asked to stand with your feet together, arms folded across your chest, and your eyes closed. If this position causes you to sway or lose your balance, it indicates that there may be a problem within your vestibular system. Most healthy individuals younger than 70 years old can maintain this pose for 30 seconds.

• Tandem walking involves walking heel to toe for 10 steps while your eyes are open and with your arms folded across your chest. The test is typically repeated three times (for a total of 30 steps), and most healthy individuals can walk a minimum of 10 steps without sidestepping. Sidestepping means you step to one side or the other rather than heel to toe. Not being able to walk 10 steps heel to toe without sidestepping indicates a problem with your vestibular system. A variation of this test is the figure eight tandem test, which requires that the muscles continuously adjust so you can maintain balance.

• You may be asked to do the turning test, in which you walk several steps with your eyes closed, turn quickly 180 degrees to the left or right, and then stop at attention. If you fall to either side, it is an indication that the weakness in the vestibular system, such as a lesion, is on that side.

• A stepping test called the Fukuda test is performed by your marching in place for at least 50 steps while your arms are extended straight out at the level of your shoulders. This test is done both with your eyes open and then with your eyes closed. People who have a problem with their vestibular system typically march slowly toward the side of the weakness. Most people don't realize they are moving away from their starting position.

CARDIOVASCULAR EXAMINATION

The doctor may also conduct a quick cardiovascular examination that includes taking your blood pressure and listening to your heart and lungs with a stethoscope. If the office is equipped with an electrocardiograph, you also may have an EKG (electrocardiogram) taken. Abnormalities or disease of the heart or blood vessels can be a cause of dizziness (see chapter 6).

EYE EXAMINATION

The eyes can reveal a great deal about a person's health. Using a few simple tests, your primary care doctor can uncover some significant clues about why you're experiencing dizziness or balance problems.

• You may be familiar with a handheld, lighted instrument called an ophthalmoscope, which doctors shine into the eyes. The ophthalmoscope allows physicians to see what's happening in the eyes and can reveal circulatory problems, diabetes, and other disorders.

• Another simple test is called the smooth pursuit test. This test is usually included as part of the electronystagmography battery of tests and is discussed in chapter 11 (see "Smooth Pursuit Test" in that chapter).

• A third test is called the vestibulo-ocular reflex test. The doctor may hold up an index finger or pencil or ask you to look at a specific object in the room. This time, however, you will slowly turn your head to one side while keeping your eyes on the object. You will repeat by turning your head to the opposite side. In this test, when you move your head to the left, your eyes move to the right. Similarly, when you turn your head to the right, your eyes move to the left. In healthy people, both the head and eye movements occur at exactly the same speed. However, if the two movements are not in synch, your vision will be blurry or you'll become dizzy. That's because there's a malfunction in your vestibulo-ocular reflex, and the likely cause is a problem in your inner ear.

Bottom Line

So far you've been introduced to the first steps you should take when trying to uncover the cause of your dizziness or balance problems. As you can see, arriving at a diagnosis for a balance disorder can involve answering many questions and undergoing various examinations and procedures. Getting to the root of a dizziness, vertigo, and/or imbalance problem can be a tricky journey, and misdiagnosis is a real possibility. However, one of the best ways you can avoid a misdiagnosis is by being an informed, involved health-care consumer. That's why we wrote this book. To become such a consumer requires that you do more than read about your balance disorder: you must also take action.

• Be as thorough as possible when completing your medical history and dizziness questionnaire. Ask family members to help you remember past medical problems or events. You may have had an experience as a young child, say a blow to the head or a bad fall off a bike or swing, that you don't remember. Perhaps you had severe ear infections and no one ever told you about them. Now is the time to ask. All of these events may be relevant to your current problem.

• Keep a journal that tracks your episodes of dizziness, vertigo, and imbalance. Write down when they happen, what precipitates each episode, how long each occurrence lasts, and if anything helps alleviate them. Don't count on being able to remember everything if you don't write it down. Once you get to the doctor's office, it's easy to forget the details, which can be so important.

PART II

WHY AM I SO DIZZY? CAUSES OF BALANCE DISORDERS

I f you are suffering with bouts of dizziness, vertigo, or disequilibrium, the inability to put a label on your condition or to
find relief from your symptoms can be frustrating, frightening,
and depressing. In this section, we hope to help alleviate those
feelings.

The information in part II can help you in two ways. If you
do not have a diagnosis, the discussion and explanation of symptoms for each condition can help you identify the type of balance
disorder you or a loved one may have. You can then take that
information, along with your journal notes, with you when you
go to a doctor. If you already have a definitive diagnosis, these
chapters can enhance your understanding of the condition,
prompt you to ask questions of your health-care practitioners,
and hopefully discover new ways to get relief.

There are literally dozens of causes of dizziness and balance
problems, and it is beyond the scope of this book to cover all of
them. In this section of the book, we discuss the more common
causes in detail. To see a list of other causes not discussed, turn to
appendix B.

4

Common Inner Ear Disorders

The inner ear is usually the first place a knowledgeable health-care practitioner looks when someone has a complaint of dizziness, vertigo, or feeling off-balance. Indeed, balance disorders that affect the inner ear are the ones physicians see most often: an estimated 40 to 45 percent of complaints of balance disorders are related to the inner ear.

In this chapter we look at the most common disorders of the inner ear that are responsible for dizziness, vertigo, and/or balance problems, including benign paroxysmal positional vertigo, Ménière's disease, recurrent vestibulopathy, and motion sickness. (Less common but still important inner ear disorders—labyrinthitis, perilymphatic fistula, ear infections, ear trauma, cholesteatoma, and otosclerosis—are covered in the next chapter.)

When you read through the conditions in this chapter, you will encounter the names of various tests used during diagnosis. You can find more information about any of these tests in chapters 3 ("Getting a Diagnosis: The First Steps") and 11 ("What to Expect If You Need Special Tests").

Benign Paroxysmal Positional Vertigo

If you've ever heard people say "She has rocks in her head," they would be right. In fact, everyone has rocks in her or his head, or, to be more accurate, ear rocks (or otoliths) in the inner ear. Usually these rocks are attached to a gelatin-like substance in the saccule and utricle. However, when these minute calcium carbonate rocks become dislodged, they can get stuck elsewhere in the inner ear and cause a condition known as benign paroxysmal positional vertigo (BPPV). Symptoms include dizziness, vertigo, disequilibrium, and nausea. Up to 25 percent of people who suffer with a vestibular disorder have BPPV.

WHO GETS BPPV?

Benign paroxysmal positional vertigo can affect people of any age, including young children, although it is more common among older individuals, like Josephine.

Everyone admired 68-year-old Josephine for her boundless energy. This retired paralegal filled her days doing volunteer work with disadvantaged children and delivering meals to shut-ins and found time to go dancing several nights a week.

One Monday morning she rolled over and sat up in bed, and seconds later a blast of severe vertigo overtook her. She tumbled off the bed and collapsed onto the floor. The episode of violent whirling lasted about 25 to 30 seconds, and then subsided. She didn't think too much of it, and chalked it up to staying up too late the night before at a dance party.

A week later, another severe vertigo episode occurred, this time while she was reaching up to remove a lunch tray from a tall cart at the volunteer center. The tray went crashing to the floor, and Josephine grabbed onto a chair as she sank to the ground. This time she felt a wave of nausea and she became worried, so she made an appointment with her doctor.

After undergoing a general physical examination, including a neurological exam and an electrocardiogram, the only thing that showed up was mildly elevated blood pressure. On her medical history, she reported that she occasionally felt slightly dizzy when getting up from a lying or seated position, and that these episodes had been happening for more than a decade.

On her dizziness questionnaire, Josephine reported that she didn't experience any ringing in her ears, hearing problems, ear infections, ear pain, or vision problems. The clue to her current problem was *when* the episodes occurred: when her head changed position with respect to gravity. That is, she was okay when she turned her head side to side, but when she went from a prone to a sitting position or when she tilted her head to look up, vertigo hit.

Her general practitioner suspected benign paroxysmal positional vertigo:

- Benign, because it is not a life-threatening condition
- Paroxysmal, because it happens suddenly and lasts only a short time
- Positional, because it occurs when the head's position is quickly changed

To help confirm the diagnosis, Josephine's doctor referred her to me. I conducted a general examination and then did a Dix-Hallpike test and other positional tests. I concluded that Josephine did indeed have BPPV, and I explained to her that in many cases, BPPV disappears spontaneously in a few days to a few months. It is, however, a treatable condition and responds quickly to positioning maneuvers in more than 80 percent of patients (see "How to Treat BPPV" below).

CAUSES AND TRIGGERS

The cause of BPPV is unknown in about 50 percent of cases. In the remaining population, a head injury or head trauma is a common cause, especially among people younger than 50 years. Among older individuals, like Josephine, a dysfunction or degeneration of the vestibular system due to aging is the usual culprit. In some people, an infection of the gastrointestinal or respiratory tract, an acute viral infection, high blood pressure, heart problems, or brain dysfunction can cause the ear rocks to float into one of the semicircular canals. (The posterior semicircular canal is affected more than 90 percent of the time in BPPV; the other two canals are much less involved.) When this happens, the canal, which is a rotation sensor (see chapter 1), is tricked into acting like a gravity sensor, and conflicting signals are sent to the brain. The result is vertigo.

Another, similar theory about what causes BPPV is that cellular "garbage" accumulates in the posterior semicircular canal and causes the pressure in the inner ear to change, resulting in vertigo. This debris eventually dissolves, and, when it does, the vertigo episodes stop. It can take six months or more for the debris to disappear.

DIAGNOSIS

Generally, doctors consider four criteria when making a diagnosis of BPPV:

- The vertigo episodes last 60 seconds or less.
- There is a three-to-five second delay between when the head is placed in the offending position and the onset of vertigo. For example, if you sit up from a lying position, as when you are getting up in the morning, and immediately stand up, vertigo may hit as you are rising. This can cause you to fall.

- The doctor or technician observes rotational eye movements (nystagmus) on the physical exam or when electronystagmography testing is done.
- The severity of the vertigo episodes decreases with each attack. This occurs because the reflexes involved in each attack become tired or fatigued each time an attack occurs and lessens the symptoms.

Often, a diagnosis can be reached on the basis of the medical history, answers on the dizziness questionnaire, physical examination, and electronystagmography test results. In some cases, doctors also conduct an audiogram if there is evidence of a hearing problem, an MRI scan if there is a possibility of a brain tumor or stroke, or a rotary chair test if the diagnosis is questionable. Although BPPV usually is confined to one ear, it can occur in both, which makes diagnosis more challenging.

HOW TO TREAT BPPV

If you are diagnosed with BPPV, your doctor may tell you that it is self-limiting, which means the symptoms typically disappear within six months of the first episode. In about 25 percent of cases, symptoms persist for longer than one year. Approximately 30 percent of the people who have one episode of BPPV have a recurrence within one year. Unfortunately, when repeat attacks will occur is unpredictable.

The good news for Josephine and for many others who have BPPV is that there are several simple, very effective maneuvers that can be done to reduce or eliminate symptoms. In Josephine's case, we did the Epley maneuver, which eliminated her symptoms. A detailed explanation of this and other maneuvers, one of which you can do at home, is found in chapter 12. In rare cases in which symptoms do not subside or respond to exercises, surgical intervention is needed. See chapter 14 for more details on a surgical procedure that can eliminate BPPV.

BENIGN PAROXYSMAL VERTIGO OF CHILDHOOD

BPV

In children, a condition known as benign paroxysmal vertigo of childhood (BPV, not to be confused with BPPV) can occur. It usually first appears in children who are 3 to 4 years of age, but it may manifest as late as 8 or 9 years. Each vertigo episode typically lasts a few seconds or minutes and is accompanied by nausea, sweating, paleness, and sometimes vomiting, but there is no *No* headache or change in consciousness. Another feature of this disorder is a strong tendency for the affected children to have a history of motion sickness.

Many experts believe there is an association between this disorder and migraine, because more than 50 percent of children with this condition subsequently develop migraine in later years and they often have a family history of migraine. Because the episodes are transient and brief, no treatment is usually needed. Some children, however, have frequent attacks (two or more a week) and can be helped if they eliminate foods that are known to trigger migraine (see chapter 13). The attacks usually occur for two to three years and then disappear when the children reach puberty.

Ménière's Disease

In 1861, a French physician named Prosper Ménière first described the inner ear disease that today affects more than 2.5 million people in the United States. Ménière's disease affects both the young and old, but it usually first appears between ages 30 and 50, a time when most people are in the full swing of raising a family, pursuing a career, and living a very active life. For about two-thirds of people with the disorder, various treatments and lifestyle changes make it possible to continue to live such a life. Some, in fact, don't require any treatment at all. For the remaining third, however, Ménière's disease can be significantly or completely disabling. *for 1/3*

VERONICA'S STORY

Veronica, a 45-year-old mother of two, says she will never forget her first attack of vertigo. "I was asleep, and a violent sensation of whirling woke me up," she says. "I was nauseous and knew I had to vomit, but I couldn't even move, the whirling was so bad. I remember calling for my kids, and they came running into my room to help me. I finally managed to crawl on my hands and knees to the bathroom and got sick. After about an hour I began to feel better."

A few weeks prior to her vertigo episode, Veronica had been experiencing a sensation of fullness in her left ear for two or three days. She noticed that sounds seemed distant in that ear, and there was constant humming in the background. She thought she might have gotten water in her ear while showering, and when the humming and hearing change went away, she didn't think any more about it.

After her vertigo episode, Veronica felt tired for several days. A few days later she felt normal again, and again she put the incident out of her mind. But six months later, she experienced another vertigo episode that lasted about an hour, and this time she came to see me the following day.

Veronica's case is a classic example of Ménière's disease. Repeat episodes of severe vertigo that typically last about one hour or more but less than a day is a typical sign. Nausea and vomiting usually accompany the whirling sensation as well. Most people also experience ringing, buzzing, or roaring in the ear (about 75 percent of Ménière's patients have the disease in one ear only) that may or may not be accompanied by a feeling of pressure or fullness in the affected ear. After the vertigo subsides, many people feel tired for several hours.

CAUSES AND TRIGGERS OF MÉNIÈRE'S DISEASE

Ménière's disease is caused by the accumulation of endolymph fluid in the inner ear. This fluid buildup produces pressure in the inner ear chamber, which causes interference with balance and hearing. This explanation is what gives Ménière's disease its other name— endolymphic hydrops, with *hydrops* meaning "fluid accumulation."

Experts are not certain why this abnormal abundance of fluid occurs. Normally, the fluids in the inner ear are constantly produced and absorbed by the inner ear system, thus maintaining a proper balance. Endolymphic hydrops is the result of either overproduction or underabsorption of the fluid, and the trigger for either of these two situations is not always known. Some of the factors believed to cause or contribute to the development of Ménière's include a genetic predisposition (there's some evidence that it runs in families), a viral infection, degeneration of the inner ear, a head injury, drug toxicity, allergies, syphilis (some people with syphilis develop Ménière's disease later in life), and autoimmune disorders. In about 40 percent of the cases, no definite cause is found.

Physical or emotional stress seems to be significantly associated with attacks of Ménière 's disease. Stress both causes the episodes and is the result of having them. Certainly, people who have Ménière's disease often live in fear of having an attack at any time, and this fear can place a great deal of stress on their lives, which can worsen their condition. The exact role of stress in Ménière's disease is still under investigation.

DIAGNOSING MÉNIÈRE'S DISEASE

No single test has been devised that can identify a case of Ménière's disease. That's one reason why it's important that you explain all the accompanying sensations and symptoms that occurred around the time of or with the vertigo when you see your doctor. The tests your doctor performs are geared to rule out other conditions characterized by vertigo, including benign paroxysmal positional vertigo, perilymph fistula, migraine, and vestibular neuronitis, among others.

Veronica underwent a physical and neurological examination, as well as balance testing, and everything was normal. This is not unusual; once the vertigo episode is over, signs of the condition are hard to find. Her electronystagmography results showed reduced vestibular response in her left ear.

She was also given an audiogram, and it showed a low-frequency hearing loss in her left ear that returned to normal in middle and high frequencies. This is a characteristic of Ménière's disease. While hearing loss associated with most other conditions first appears in the high frequencies, in Ménière's it's the opposite. Thus I diagnosed Ménière's disease on the basis of Veronica's history and the results of her audiogram.

UNPREDICTABILITY

One frustrating and frightening thing about Ménière's disease is its unpredictability: people don't know when the next attack will strike. Some people experience episodes of vertigo at regular intervals, say, every few days, once a week, or every few weeks. Others go for months without an attack. Some people have minor incidents of disequilibrium and dizziness that last a few minutes between major attacks. Fortunately, some people have one severe episode and symptoms never return.

Another unpredictable feature of Ménière's disease is that occasionally, noise in the ears, a feeling of pressure in the ear, and hearing loss occur without vertigo. This condition is known as cochlear Ménière's disease. Yet a third type of Ménière's disease is vestibular Ménière's disease, which is characterized solely by vertigo and a sensation of fullness in the ear. Your doctor may tell you you have one of these forms of Ménière's disease. Because all forms of Ménière's disease are treated similarly, we are including all three forms when we talk about Ménière's disease in this book.

TREATMENT: FIRST CHOICE

The goal of treatment of Ménière's disease is to improve an individual's quality of life, which means stopping the vertigo and preventing hearing loss. To accomplish these goals, it's necessary to improve the metabolism of the inner ear, either via dietary approaches, drugs (diuretics are used most often along with dietary recommendations), or surgery. (See chapters 13 and 14 for more details on dietary and surgical approaches.)

My first choice of treatment approach is one that people can follow easily at home. It includes:

- Consuming a low-salt diet. Salt causes the retention of fluids throughout the body; therefore a low-salt diet can help reduce the amount of fluid that accumulates in the inner ear.
- Taking a diuretic. Diuretics, or water pills, help the kidneys excrete excess fluid. Water pills are often prescribed along with a low-salt diet to help decrease the pressure caused by the buildup of fluid in the inner ear. The three most effective diuretics are acetazolamide (Dazamide and Diamox), hydrochlorothiazide/triamtene (Dyazide), and hydrochloro-thiazide (Hydrodiuril). Side effects may include rash, muscle cramps, weakness, dizziness, and diarrhea.
- Avoiding caffeine, alcohol, and significant amounts of sugar. Caffeine can reduce blood circulation in the inner ear, alcohol in excess can cause dizziness; and sugar may cause fluctuations in fluid levels in the inner ear.
- Undergoing a stress management program. Although the exact role of stress in Ménière's disease is not known, stress is known to hinder healing and recovery from illness in general; plus anxiety is a cause of dizziness.
- Stopping smoking. Nicotine and other smoking by-products reduce the inner ear circulation and interfere with proper inner ear function.

These were the recommendations I prescribed for Veronica. I closely followed her progress for the next six months, and during that time she didn't experience any more vertigo episodes, and the humming and feeling of fullness in her ear disappeared.

At six months, I recommended that Veronica stop taking the diuretics. Generally, if patients have been free of vertigo episodes for six months while following the diet and taking a diuretic, I stop the drug to see how the patients will do on their own. In Veronica's case, she stopped the diuretic at six months and felt fine. She has regained control of her life and has not required any additional interventions.

DRUG TREATMENT

Besides diuretics, drugs that can help reduce vertigo, such as antihistamines, antiemetics, or sedatives, may be prescribed. However, because these medications can hinder the brain's ability to compensate and thus lengthen recovery time, they are generally recommended only for occasional use when vertigo attacks are causing a significant impact on a person's lifestyle.

If your health-care practitioner does prescribe drugs to help lessen the severity of the symptoms associated with vertigo attacks, he or she may recommend one of the following:

- Meclizine (Antivert) is an antihistamine that helps prevent nausea and vomiting. It is usually recommended for milder vertigo attacks. Common side effects include blurry vision, dry mouth, drowsiness, and fatigue. You should not take meclizine if you have asthma, prostate hypertrophy, pulmonary disease, or untreated glaucoma. It is safe for use during pregnancy.

- Promethazine (Anergan, Antinaus, Pentazine, Phenerzine, and Phenergan, among others), also an antihistamine, is for severe vertigo episodes accompanied by nausea and vomiting. It is used only for acute attacks; it cannot prevent recurrent episodes. The most significant side effect is drowsiness. It is available as a tablet or suppository.

- Prochlorperazine (Compazine) or metoclopramide (Maxolon, Octamide, and Reglan), are antiemetics (antinausea/

antivomiting) that can be taken along with meclizine for better control of symptoms. Side effects can include blurry vision, drowsiness, dizziness, lightheadedness, dry mouth, constipation, and weight gain. They are available as a tablet or suppository or by injection by your doctor.

- Droperidol (Inapsine) is a sedative that is available as an injection, intravenously, or as a sublingual (under the tongue) drop. It is typically given in an emergency room or hospital setting. Droperidol is effective against acute attacks and can last as long as 24 hours. Side effects include drowsiness and hypotension. Do not take this drug if you have kidney or liver disease.

ROLE OF VESTIBULAR REHABILITATION THERAPY

As a rule, vestibular rehabilitation is not effective in the management of vertigo attacks associated with Ménière's disease. However, some people who have Ménière's disease, especially older individuals, experience recurring problems with balance as part of the disease. For example, after episodes of vertigo, some people don't recover their prior level of balance control and experience lingering balance difficulties such as unsteadiness when getting out of bed or when walking on uneven surfaces. For these people, vestibular rehabilitation therapy can be very effective in helping them regain a better quality of life (see chapter 12, "Vestibular Rehabilitation and Other Physical Therapies").

SURGERY FOR MÉNIÈRE'S DISEASE

In less than one-third of the cases of Ménière's disease, diet, stress management, and diuretics aren't effective. Stephen, a 54-year-old attorney, had all the classic symptoms of Ménière's disease. Unlike Veronica, however, he was having vertigo attacks every few weeks. At first we tried dietary changes, diuretics, and a stress management program (meditation), but the vertigo episodes continued. The unpredictability of the attacks affected his performance in court and with clients, and he opted for a surgical procedure called vestibular neurectomy (see chapter 14, "Surgical and Medical Procedures").

Since his surgery, Stephen has enjoyed a vertigo-free life. He has even been able to continue to participate in one of his lifelong passions—sailing—without any problems with dizziness or disequilibrium.

Vestibular rehabilitation after vestibular neurectomy is usually not necessary when the patient leads a relatively active life, as the brain compensates virtually spontaneously. Elderly patients, however, usually require several sessions of therapy to assist in brain compensation. (Read more about vestibular rehabilitation therapy in chapter 12.)

BILATERAL MÉNIÈRE'S DISEASE

In 20 to 30 percent of people who have Ménière's disease, both ears are affected. This was the case for Lorraine, a 62-year-old semiretired librarian who had been living with Ménière's disease in her right ear for about ten years. She had some hearing loss in that ear as well.

After a decade of having learned to live and cope with Ménière's disease in one ear, Lorraine began experiencing a loud sound in her left ear and, most frightening of all, drop attacks. Drop attacks are episodes of vertigo that are so severe and sudden that, without warning, you instantly lose all control and fall to the ground. Such attacks can be extremely dangerous and result in fractures.

Lorraine made an appointment to see me immediately, and she came in for testing. Even though her tests indicated that only her right ear had hearing loss and vestibular weakness, her symptoms told us they were coming from her left ear. Lorraine now realized that her disease was taking control of her life, and she looked at some surgical options.

We chose endolymphatic sac decompression, and the surgery was a success. Today she no longer has drop attacks, and she has maintained her presurgical level of hearing. If the procedure had not been successful, we could have chosen a more radical procedure, which is usually reserved for people who don't respond to less aggressive procedures and/or who have more severe symptoms. For details on surgical procedures for Ménière's disease, see chapter 14.

Recurrent Vestibulopathy

When trying to uncover the cause of dizziness or a balance problem, doctors often arrive at their diagnosis by excluding a long list of other disorders before arriving at the apparent one. When a doctor is confronted with a possible case of recurrent vestibulopathy, one of the main disorders he or she excludes is Ménière's disease, because these two conditions resemble each other in many ways. The good news about recurrent vestibulopathy, however, is that unlike Ménière's disease, it is much more likely to improve with treatment.

Recurrent vestibulopathy, which is also known as benign recurrent vertigo or vestibular Ménière's disease, is the most common vestibular syndrome caused by migraine. It is characterized by multiple episodes of vertigo that typically last up to 20 minutes, although some may last longer. These episodes are accompanied by nausea and vomiting, and then are usually followed by disequilibrium that lasts up to a few days. Ringing in the ears may occur, but there is no hearing loss. William's case is typical.

WILLIAM'S STORY

William, a 48-year-old insurance salesman, had become increasingly concerned about several severe episodes of vertigo he had experienced over two years. His most recent attack—his fourth—had occurred one week before he came into my office. He described each event as follows: a severe whirling sensation that lasted about 20 to 30 minutes, accompanied by nausea and vomiting. Each attack sent him to bed, where he had to stay for five to six hours until he felt stable enough to get up. After the vertigo subsided, he would have some trouble keeping his balance for the next few days; then he would recover fully. Six or eight months would go by before he would have another episode. In between, he felt fine.

DIAGNOSIS

Because recurrent vestibulopathy is a diagnosis of exclusion and the cause is unknown, we considered other conditions characterized by recurrent vertigo, such as benign paroxysmal positional vertigo and other inner ear disorders, as well as various cardiovascular, seizure, and panic disorders. William's physical examination was normal, as were his positional testing, caloric test, audiogram, and MRI.

William's history and dizziness questionnaire revealed that each vertigo episode was not accompanied by any hearing loss, ringing in the ears, fullness in the ears, vision problems, numbness, or weakness. He didn't suffer from migraines, and he had no history of head or ear trauma or neurological disorders, such as multiple sclerosis or Parkinson's disease. On the basis of these findings, we arrived at a diagnosis of recurrent vestibulopathy.

TREATMENT

Your first line of treatment for recurrent vestibulopathy is dietary changes and an allergy workup to help avoid allergic triggers (food and inhalants) (see chapter 13, "Treating Dizziness with Diet," for more information). These measures can help prevent future attacks. To relieve symptoms of vertigo, nausea, and vomiting when they occur (and not as a preventive measure), antiemetic (antinausea/antivomiting) drugs or an antihistamine are recommended.

- Prochlorperazine (Compazine) or metoclopramide (Maxolon, Octamide, and Reglan) are antiemetics (antinausea /vomiting) and are available as tablets and suppositories. You will likely need the suppository, especially if you experience vomiting. Side effects can include blurry vision, drowsiness, dizziness, lightheadedness, dry mouth, constipation, and weight gain.
- Promethazine (Anergan, Antinaus, Pentazine, Phenerzine, and Phenergan, among others) is an antihistamine used to treat acute, severe vertigo episodes accompanied by nausea and vomiting. It cannot prevent recurrent episodes. The most significant side effect is drowsiness. It is available as a tablet and suppository.

Motion Sickness

For many people, young and old alike, the thought of taking a road trip in a car or bus or going out into the bay or ocean on a cabin cruiser, sail boat, or cruise ship makes them turn green, and not with envy. For these individuals, motion sickness, characterized by dizziness, queasy stomach, nausea, and vomiting, takes any enjoyment out of such trips.

WHY PEOPLE GET MOTION SICKNESS

Motion sickness is the result of mismatched signals between what your eyes see, what your inner ear senses, and how the brain interprets the information. For example, say you're in the cabin of a boat that's rocking gently with the waves. You look across the room and everything appears to be upright, but the gravity sensors in your inner ear and the pressure sensors in the bottom of your feet are shouting "This room is tilting!" Thus your eyes tell your brain one thing and your ears and feet tell it another; this causes confusion. The result is dizziness, nausea, and/or vomiting.

A similar situation exists if you try to read in a moving vehicle. Your inner ears and your skin receptors tell you that you're moving, but your eyes are looking at a newspaper that isn't. Unless your brain can unscramble the mixed signals, you'll likely begin to feel dizzy, queasy, and sick to your stomach.

CAUSES

Naturally, not everyone gets motion sickness, so why are some people more susceptible than others? Genetics appears to play a role, but so do hormones. Studies show that people who get motion sickness secrete greater amounts of epinephrine and norepinephrine (stress hormones) than people who don't experience this disorder. The high levels of stress hormones cause a rise in the hormone vasopressin, which triggers muscle contractions in the stomach, which result in vomiting.

Some people experience motion sickness even if they are standing or sitting perfectly still and they are viewing objects that are moving. This type of disorder, called pure optokinetic motion sickness, would only be apparent if you were, say, in a theater with a panoramic screen on which there were constantly moving images.

HOW TO PREVENT AND TREAT MOTION SICKNESS

In today's fast-moving society, being susceptible to motion sickness can be a challenge, but not one that can't be met. Here are some tips on how to prevent the symptoms of motion sickness.

- Position yourself in the place with the least amount of movement. This works for planes and boats, but not for cars. In planes, get an aisle seat over the wings; in a boat, stay in the middle rather than at the front or sides.

• Face the direction in which you are traveling. Avoid sitting backward in your seat or in a seat that faces backward (common on trains).

• Look out and ahead. When in a car, look out the window at things that are far away. In a boat, focus on the horizon. In a plane, look out the window.

• Don't read or look at maps or any type of printed materials while in motion.

• Before you travel, either don't eat or eat a light meal only. Avoid fats and fried or spicy foods. Low-fat carbohydrates, such as saltines, bagels, whole grain cereals, or pretzels, are a good choice. While traveling, eat several small meals rather than a few large ones.

• When riding in a car, sit in the front seat and look out the front window, not the side.

• Get fresh air. In a car, open the window or use the air conditioning. In a plane, allow the air vents to blow on you.

• Try exercises that can help you deal with mismatched stimuli (see chapter 12).

• Both over-the-counter and prescription medications are available to help reduce or avoid motion sickness. They include:

    • Meclizine (prescription drug Antivert and over-the-counter drugs Bonine and Dramamine II). This drug reaches its maximum effectiveness seven to nine hours after you take it, so schedule your dose accordingly when you plan to travel. The most common side effects are blurry vision, dry mouth, drowsiness, and fatigue. Do not take meclizine if you plan to drive. Also avoid meclizine if you have asthma, pulmonary disease, prostate hypertrophy, or untreated glaucoma. It is safe to use during pregnancy, but always check with your obstetrician first.

    • Scopolamine (the prescription drug Transderm Scop). This drug is especially helpful for long-term travel, such as a cruise, because it comes in a transdermal patch, which you wear on your skin for three days. After three days, you remove the old patch and apply a new one. Because it takes four to eight hours for the drug's effects to become apparent, you should put the patch on at least that much time before you leave on your trip. The most common side effects are drowsiness and dry mouth. On rare occasions, people experience urinary retention, amnesia, disorientation, and hallucinations. Thus, scopolamine should not be used by children or the elderly. Avoid scopolamine if you have glaucoma or an enlarged prostate.

Bottom Line

If you have one of the more common inner ear conditions discussed in this chapter, you're not alone: millions of Americans struggle with these problems every day. As you've seen here, there are steps you can take today to help regain control of your life and rid yourself of dizziness or balance problems. If you think you have a condition that warrants medical attention, see a knowledgeable physician and bring your journal and dizziness questionnaire with you on your first visit. Also look at the treatment options discussed in chapters 12 through 15 so you'll be more informed about these approaches when you see your doctor.

5

Other Inner Ear Disorders

Although the inner ear disorders discussed in this chapter may not be as common as those we explored in the previous chapter, we can guarantee they are of great significance if you are the individual experiencing them. That's why we decided to take a closer look at labyrinthitis, vestibular neuronitis, perilymphatic fistula, cholesteatoma, otosclerosis, and height dizziness/vertigo in this chapter.

When you read through the conditions in this chapter, you will encounter the names of various tests used during diagnosis. You can find more information about any of these tests in chapters 3 ("Getting a Diagnosis: The First Steps") and 11 ("What to Expect If You Need Special Tests").

Labyrinthitis and Vestibular Neuronitis

When most people think about ear infections, they typically associate them with infants and young children, many of whom seem to be constantly plagued with these often painful conditions. The type of ear infections that usually affect children (and some adults) involve the middle ear and are discussed below in "Other Ear Infections." Here we discuss two closely related conditions which involve infection of the inner ear and that cause vertigo and disequilibrium:

- Labyrinthitis, infection or inflammation of the inner ear
- Vestibular neuronitis (also called vestibular neuritis), infection or inflammation of the vestibular nerve, which carries signals from the inner ear to the brain

About 10 percent of people who have a vestibular disorder suffer with labyrinthitis or vestibular neuronitis.

SIMILAR YET DIFFERENT

The terms *labyrinthitis* and *vestibular neuronitis* are often used interchangeably, and many doctors believe they are basically the same condition, with the only difference being the location of the infection or inflammation. One significant difference doctors must identify, however, is whether the cause of the labyrinthitis or vestibular neuronitis is viral or bacterial. If the cause is bacterial, antibiotic treatment should begin immediately, as a bacterial infection is much more serious than a viral one. That being said, let's look at these two conditions.

Labyrinthitis is a condition in which there is inflammation *(-itis)* of the labyrinth, the system in the inner ear that consists of the cochlea, the semicircular canals, and the surrounding structures. It is the most common complication of otitis media, an infection of the middle ear. A viral infection is the most common cause of labyrinthitis; influenza, herpes, measles, hepatitis, adenovirus, polio, coxsackie, Epstein-Barr, and mumps have all been found to be associated with this disease.

Vestibular neuronitis involves inflammation of the vestibular nerve, and usually develops shortly after a viral infection, most often an upper respiratory tract infection or a cold. The infection attacks the vestibular nerve and causes it to become inflamed, which then results in inaccurate signals being sent to the brain.

Bacterial Labyrinthitis. In a minority of cases, labyrinthitis is caused by a bacterial infection. If bacteria get into the labyrinth, they can cause damage in several ways. When the bacteria infect the middle ear or the bone that surrounds the inner ear, toxins are produced that cause the cochlea, the vestibular system, or both to become inflamed. This type of labyrinthitis is called serous labyrinthitis and is usually caused by an untreated chronic middle ear infection. Constant imbalance and dizziness are classic symptoms.

If the bacteria invade the labyrinth, they cause suppurative labyrinthitis. The bacteria that cause this type of bacterial labyrinthitis typically enter the inner ear of people who have bacterial meningitis, which is an inflammation of the covering that protects the brain. Suppurative labyrinthitis can also be caused by bacteria that enter the inner ear through an injury, as occurs in perilymphatic fistula (see below). Again, constant imbalance and dizziness are common symptoms.

Hearing loss may occur in cases of bacterial labyrinthitis. Left untreated, the infection can result in a brain abscess, meningitis, or deafness.

Viral Labyrinthitis and Vestibular Neuronitis. In cases of both viral labyrinthitis and vestibular neuronitis, experts believe the virus enters the inner ear through the upper airway or the blood stream. In addition to the viral infections already named, other viruses could be involved in these ear diseases, but doctors cannot identify them because it isn't possible to collect tissue samples from the inner ear without damaging the labyrinth.

In most cases of viral labyrinthitis, symptoms come on suddenly. If the infection affects the cochlea, you can expect to experience some hearing loss and ringing in the ears, although not everyone gets these symptoms. If the virus reaches the vestibular system, dizziness, severe vertigo with nausea and vomiting, and imbalance can occur. Because the entire inner ear is so small, the infection nearly always affects both hearing and balance.

The vertigo episode can last as long as 48 hours, and then be followed by two to seven days of severe disequilibrium along with intermittent attacks of vertigo that are triggered by certain movements. The disequilibrium typically subsides slowly over the next few weeks as do the episodes of vertigo. However, it could take as long as six months for the symptoms to disappear completely.

Vestibular neuronitis differs slightly from viral labyrinthitis in that there is no hearing loss. Both labyrinthitis and vestibular neuronitis are self-limiting conditions; this is fortunate because there are no effective treatments for these diseases. Antibiotics, which can be given for bacterial labyrinthitis, are not effective against viruses. However, medications can be given to treat the symptoms of nausea, vomiting, and dizziness (see "Treatment" below). About 50 percent of the people affected recover completely while the rest experience significant improvement.

DIAGNOSIS

Because a bacterial infection of the inner ear can result in serious consequences, it's important that you describe your symptoms and any precipitating events as accurately as possible so your doctor can better arrive at a correct diagnosis as soon as possible. If a bacterial infection is identified, antibiotic therapy can begin.

If there are no signs of a bacterial infection and if you or a close family member recently experienced a viral infection, your doctor will suspect a viral cause for your inner ear infection. If you've recently had a head injury, tell your doctor, as a blow to the head can damage the inner ear and cause symptoms that mimic those of an inner ear infection.

TREATMENT

As we mentioned, bacterial labyrinthitis should be treated immediately with antibiotics to avoid serious complications. Most cases of labyrinthitis and vestibular neuronitis have a viral cause, however, and antibiotics are ineffective against viruses. Viral cases are self-limiting, and so most patients can expect to experience a reduction in symptoms after a week or two, with full recovery taking several months. Treatment of viral labyrinthitis and vestibular neuronitis may include use of the following drugs, although these medications may also delay recovery:

- Antiemetic (antinausea/antivomiting) drugs prochlorperazine (Compazine) and metoclopramide (Maxolon, Octamide, and Reglan) are available as tablets and suppositories. Use the suppositories if you are experiencing vomiting. Side effects of these drugs include blurry vision, drowsiness, dizziness, light-headedness, weight gain, dry mouth, and constipation.
- Corticosteroids (methylprednisolone [Medrol], prednisone [Deltasone], and dexamethasone [Decadron]) are sometimes prescribed for short-term use to help reduce inflammation in the inner ear and control hearing loss. Common side effects include acne, indigestion, nausea, vomiting, headache, insomnia, dizziness, increased appetite, weight gain, and swollen feet and legs. These drugs are available in tablet, capsule, and liquid forms. Avoid the use of corticosteroids if you have tuberculosis, herpes infection of the eyes, peptic ulcer disease, or a systemic fungal infection.
- Promethazine (Anergan, Antinaus, Pentazine, Phenerzine, Phenergan, and others) helps suppress dizziness, nausea, and vomiting. It is useful for acute attacks but not as a preventive measure. Promethazine is effective within 1 to 2 hours of

ingestion, and its effects last for up to 12 hours. The most common side effect is drowsiness.

Vestibular rehabilitation is recommended during the months of recovery to help individuals manage transitory dizziness and problems with balance. Read more about vestibular rehabilitation therapy in chapter 12.

Other Ear Infections

In addition to vestibular neuronitis, viral labyrinthitis, and bacterial labyrinthitis, other types of ear infections can affect balance. Middle ear infection (acute otitis media), fluid in the middle ear (serous otitis), and a hole in the eardrum that may secrete fluid (chronic otitis media) cause pain and swelling and sometimes dizziness, balance problems, and hearing loss. Infants and toddlers who are affected with ear infections usually pull or poke at their ears. Other indications include vomiting, drainage from the ear, decreased appetite, fever, and excessive fussiness and crying. Older children and adults will often complain about dizziness and pain, pressure, fullness, and/or popping in the ear. Fever and ear drainage are often present as well. Antibiotics are typically prescribed for these infections.

Some middle ear infections become chronic, and although they are usually painless, they are associated with a foul-smelling discharge from the ear and hearing loss, and occasionally ringing in the ears, dizziness, and facial weakness. This is a serious condition that usually requires surgical removal of the infected portion of the middle ear.

Perilymphatic Fistula

A perilymphatic fistula is a tear or break in one or both of the tiny, thin interfaces—the oval window and round window—that lie between the middle and inner ears. This break leads to difficulties with balance, dizziness, and hearing.

When intact, the oval and round windows prevent the fluid from the inner ear from leaking into the middle ear. They also do not allow changes in air pressure in the middle ear (as when your ears "pop" when ascending or descending in an airplane) to affect the inner ear. The presence of a fistula thus changes the balance of fluids and pressure between these two parts of the ear; this in turn stimulates the inner ear and results in symptoms.

HOW TO RECOGNIZE PERILYMPHATIC FISTULA

Symptoms of perilymphatic fistula can vary a great deal; this makes it a difficult condition to diagnose. Generally, the most common symptoms include dizziness, disequilibrium (which can be intermittent or chronic), hearing loss (often fluctuating, but it may be constant), ringing in the ears, nausea, and vomiting. You may also experience vertigo, especially when you cough, sneeze, lift, bend over, or strain during defecation. Episodes of vertigo may last only seconds or as long as several hours. The severity of symptoms can change depending on changes in the weather, air pressure, and altitude (especially if you are flying, taking a high-rise elevator, or traveling at high elevations), as well as with physical activity.

CAUSES AND TRIGGERS

The most common cause of a perilymphatic fistula is some type of head trauma, such as whiplash from an automobile accident, a sports-related injury, an open hand slap to the ear, or a direct blow to the head. They also can be caused by a rapid change in air pressure, which can occur when scuba diving or when a plane takes a steep dive or ascent, or by intense straining, such as during childbirth or weight lifting. In a small percentage of cases there is a congenital inner ear abnormality.

DIAGNOSIS

Perilymphatic fistula can be difficult to diagnose because symptoms can vary a great deal. This makes a patient's history, especially any type of head injury, extremely important in the diagnostic process.

Gavin is a 27-year-old electrician who first went to see his primary care doctor complaining of lightheadedness and dizziness that got worse when he moved his head rapidly. He had been experiencing these sensations daily for more than a month, and they were accompanied by some hearing loss and occasional ringing in his ears. Gavin noted that the dizziness got worse when he had to bend over, and this was making it difficult for him to work.

Gavin told his doctor that the symptoms had begun the day after he had hit his head hard on the ground during a game of tag football. Because he hadn't lost consciousness or felt unbalanced after the hit, he hadn't thought the fall was important. When he realized that the fall might be responsible for his dizziness and other symptoms, he procrastinated until they affected his ability to work.

After taking his medical history and conducting a physical examination, Gavin's doctor ordered a computed tomography (CT) scan, which came back normal. The tuning fork test indicated a hearing problem in the left ear but not in the right. He then referred Gavin to me.

On the basis of Gavin's symptoms and the fact that they had started immediately after a recent head injury, I suspected either a concussion of the inner ear (labyrinth), endolymphatic hydrops (swelling of the endolymphatic compartment of the inner ear), or perilymphatic fistula. A clue that pointed to perilymphatic fistula was the fact that his symptoms were worse when he coughed, sneezed, or strained, activities that are collectively referred to as Valsalva maneuvers.

Gavin underwent the Romberg test, which was negative. An audiogram showed both conductive and sensorineural hearing loss in his left ear. When we conducted the rotary chair test, results indicated a vestibular dysfunction. The fistula test triggered nystagmus (abnormal, jerky eye movements) and dizziness when done in the left ear but not in the right, a good indication that a fistula was present. Considering all the findings, I made a diagnosis of perilymphatic fistula.

TREATMENT

The only way to make a definite diagnosis of perilymphatic fistula is to perform a procedure called a tympanotomy, which allows doctors to see if there is any damage to the oval or round membranes. Fortunately, this procedure can be avoided in most cases if the patient is willing to stay in bed for four to seven days, as inactivity and rest allow a fistula to heal in many cases. This was the avenue Gavin chose, and within a week his symptoms disappeared.

Not everyone is so lucky, however. If your symptoms are severe, if you do not respond to strict bed rest, or if your hearing loss worsens, surgery is usually required to repair the fistula by using tissue grafts.

Cholesteatoma

A cholesteatoma is a skin cyst that causes the destruction of bone in the middle ear and, rarely, in the inner ear. It is usually found along with a chronic middle ear infection (chronic otitis media), especially in people who have a history of middle ear infections. Symptoms include hearing loss and a foul-smelling intermittent or constant discharge. Dizziness, vertigo, and problems with balance occur if the destruction has reached the inner ear or if there is fistula formation or infection.

A cholesteatoma can form for several reasons.

- If the eardrum becomes perforated (punctured, a hole caused) due to trauma or chronic infection, the skin on the outer surface of the eardrum may grow through the perforation and into the middle ear.

- Heredity can be the cause. Some people are born with a tiny piece of skin that is trapped in the middle ear or, rarely, in the inner ear.
- The Eustachian tube, the canal that connects the middle ear to the back of the nose, may malfunction. This tube equalizes the pressure between the middle ear and the outer environment. If the tube fails to work properly, it causes a negative pressure in the middle ear, and over time the eardrum retracts toward the inner ear, causing the formation of a skin sac that can cause infection and bone destruction.

In all these cases, the skin cyst sheds dead skin cells, which accumulate inside the ear. As the dead cells continue to gather, the lining of the cyst produces enzymes that cause bone destruction.

HOW TO RECOGNIZE CHOLESTEATOMA

The main signs and symptoms of cholesteatoma are hearing difficulties and a foul-smelling fluid that drains from the affected ear. Others include dizziness, brief spells of vertigo, disequilibrium, and weakness on the side of the face of the affected ear.

The hearing loss occurs as the bones behind the eardrum or the ossicles (the three small bones in the middle ear used for hearing) are destroyed. If the bone over the facial nerve is damaged, facial paralysis can result. Destruction of the bones of the inner ear can lead to dizziness and further hearing loss. If left untreated, the infection can be carried by the bloodstream to the brain and cause meningitis or a brain abscess.

DIAGNOSIS

Brenda, a 35-year-old elementary school teacher, came to the office two days after she noticed a foul-smelling fluid draining from her right ear and after experiencing a brief episode of vertigo, accompanied by nausea and vomiting. She also reported that she had been having some trouble hearing in her right ear.

Brenda's physical and neurological exams were normal, and she passed the Romberg and gait tests. An audiogram showed normal hearing in her left ear but some loss of hearing in her right. Her ear examination showed a yellow discharge and a perforation in her tympanic membrane. We also did a CT scan of the temporal bone, which is the bone that contains the structures of the inner ear. A healthy inner ear should show black on a CT scan, but Brenda's was gray, which indicated an infection and cholesteatoma. Electronystagmography tests were not performed because of the infection and because such tests would be very uncomfortable in the presence of an ear infection.

TREATMENT

In Brenda's case, the cholesteatoma was relatively small, so we were able to treat her with antibiotics first to stop the infection. Surgery to remove the cholesteatoma was then performed successfully (see chapter 14, "Surgical and Medical Procedures"). The goal of treatment is to control the infection because once it is out of hand, it can cause serious brain damage.

Otosclerosis

Otosclerosis is a metabolic condition that affects the bony labyrinth and ossicles and causes hearing loss. Over time, abnormal bone growth develops, usually involving the stapes (the ossicles closest to the inner ear), and the result is conductive hearing loss. In some cases, there is damage to the sensory cells or nerves of the inner ear as well, which results in sensorineural hearing loss. Vertigo and disequilibrium are also common symptoms.

Seventy percent of the people who have otosclerosis first

notice some hearing loss between the ages of 20 and 30. Otosclerosis affects whites more than blacks, and is nearly nonexistent among Asian Americans and Native Americans. Overall, about 2 percent of the population has this ear disorder.

WHAT CAUSES OTOSCLEROSIS?

Between 50 and 70 percent of people who have otosclerosis have a family history of the disease. However, the exact cause of the disorder is not known. Some research suggests that viral infections are involved, while others say the hormonal changes that occur during pregnancy have a role. In fact, otosclerosis can accelerate during a woman's second pregnancy.

HOW TO RECOGNIZE OTOSCLEROSIS

The first sign of otosclerosis is usually an inability to hear soft sounds, and this failure may appear gradually. Although otosclerosis is usually thought of as a hearing disorder, many people also experience recurrent episodes of vertigo and disequilibrium, and in some cases, ringing in the ears.

DIAGNOSIS

Because hearing loss is the primary sign of otosclerosis, an audiogram (see chapter 11) and a tympanogram, which shows how the middle ear is able to conduct sound, are usually done and typically reveal a conductive hearing loss. Vestibular function tests such as the electronystagmography, rotary chair, and posturography are requested as needed in case of vestibular symptoms.

TREATMENT

There is no known cure for otosclerosis, but there are treatment options.

• Fluoride supplementation may slow or stop the progression of the disease. Oral doses of sodium fluoride can stabilize the hearing loss that is associated with otosclerosis in about 80 percent of the patients. The fluoride reduces the amount of bone that is absorbed, promotes the growth of new bone, and thus virtually stops any further progression of the damage. Sodium fluoride also can reduce symptoms of disequilibrium and ringing in the ears. Typically, patients take a specific dosage for about two years or until the disease has stabilized. Some people take sodium fluoride for 6 to 12 months before undergoing stapedectomy to promote healing of the affected area and help reduce any chance that the disease will progress after surgery. Side effects can include rash and gastrointestinal upset.

• If hearing loss is mild or moderate, a hearing aid that amplifies sound may be necessary. Your otologist or audiologist can help you select the most effective device for your needs.

• A surgical procedure called stapedectomy can help restore hearing loss. Like any surgical procedure, stapedectomy is associated with risks and possible complications. However, the success rates and excellent hearing results after a stapedectomy far outweigh the risks, and most patients with otosclerosis do tend to choose the surgical option

• Vestibular rehabilitation therapy is usually recommended for people who have disequilibrium with their otosclerosis to help them manage their balance.

Height Vertigo

Are you afraid of heights? Do you get dizzy when you're on a high floor of a tall building or when you peer down over the railing of a high balcony? Which came first, the fear or the dizziness?

Some people have an intense fear of heights (acrophobia) that began after they experienced a severe dizzy spell while in a height situation. Others seem to first have the fear, typically as a manifestation of anxiety and an intense fear of falling, and dizziness or vertigo is part of their phobia. This latter condition is discussed in chapter 9.

True physiological height vertigo—also known as height dizziness—is a condition that is triggered visually, and then manifested by swaying of the body, a fear of falling, and sometimes nausea. If you have height vertigo, you may experience dizziness when you look down from a tall building, rooftop, balcony, bridge, or glass-sided elevator.

WHAT CAUSES HEIGHT VERTIGO?

Physiological height vertigo is sometimes referred to as a "distance vertigo." That's because a major cause appears to be the amount of distance between the eyes and the nearest visible stationary objects. For some people, standing on the third-floor balcony and looking out over the edge to the ground below may be the defining distance; others may not be affected until they are ten or more stories high. Thus the vertigo is visually induced—determined by what an individual identifies (involuntarily) to be the distance that causes the imbalance. Added to this physical sensation of vertigo are any fears—of falling, tripping, becoming ill, or the building's collapsing—which add to the anxiety and thus the vertigo.

HOW TO PREVENT HEIGHT DIZZINESS

Avoidance of height situations is the best way to prevent height dizziness, but if you are unable to stay away from such circumstances completely, here are a few tips to help prevent the vertigo and other symptoms.

- If you are standing, make sure you are holding onto a stationary object, such as a wall, railing, or doorway. Do not hold onto an object that can move, such as a table or chair.

- Do not look at moving objects, such as clouds or cars. This increases the risk of falling because your ability to maintain a steady posture is compromised.
- Do not look through binoculars, because this restricts your field of vision while also introducing the added distraction of magnification.
- Stand with your feet firmly planted on a level surface and keep your head in line with your trunk. Avoid tilting your head.

Bottom Line

Like the more common inner ear disorders discussed in chapter 4, those explained in this chapter can throw your life into turmoil. And, because they are less common, diagnosis may be more elusive unless your health-care provider—and you—take an aggressive approach to it.

Now that you are more informed about these conditions, you're ready for action. Familiarize yourself with your treatment options as well (see chapters 12 through 15) and see a knowledgeable physician if you believe you have a medical condition that requires attention.

6

Cardiovascular and Central Nervous System Disorders

Millions of Americans—and perhaps you are among them—have medical problems that affect either the central nervous system (the brain and spinal cord) or the cardiovascular system (the heart, blood, and blood vessels). And, if you are like many of those millions, you're unaware that dizziness and problems with balance are symptoms that often appear as part of these conditions.

In previous chapters, we briefly discussed the role of the brain in balance disorders. In this chapter, we'll explore that relationship more fully. But you may be wondering what possible role the heart or the blood supply could have in maintaining balance. We'll solve that mystery for you as well.

An understanding of the relationship between cardiovascular and central nervous system conditions, and dizziness and disequilibrium is important for you for several reasons. One, if you have been diagnosed with a cardiovascular or central nervous system disorder, you may not have been told that you may experience lightheadedness, dizziness, spinning sensations, and/or problems with balance as part of your condition. If you're not aware that they are often part of these ailments, you may become frightened or anxious.

Two, sometimes these symptoms are among the first indications that you have one of these disorders. Therefore, recognizing these symptoms now may prompt you to get much-needed and timely medical attention. And three, you'll be better able to help your doctors uncover the source of your dizziness and associated symptoms if you know more about the different medical conditions of which they can be a part.

Central Nervous System Disorders

The central nervous system is literally the command center of the balance system. It's the translation and transmission station for all the signals that come in from the vestibular, visual, and proprioceptive systems. So naturally, when something goes wrong with a part of the central nervous system, there's a good chance that dizziness, vertigo, and/or disequilibrium, along with hearing problems and other associated symptoms, could result.

Here we discuss some of the more common central nervous system disorders of which lightheadedness, dizziness, balance problems, and/or vertigo may be characteristic.

ACOUSTIC NEUROMA

An acoustic neuroma is a benign (noncancerous), often slow-growing tumor that develops on the eighth cranial nerve, usually at the base of the brain where the auditory nerve leaves the skull and enters the bony structure of the inner ear. Development of an acoustic neuroma is often accompanied by balance problems and can be associated with symptoms that include vertigo, dizziness, loss of balance, ringing in the ears, hearing loss (in the affected ear), facial pain, vision problems, and headache that intensifies when lying down, coughing, sneezing, straining, or lifting.

An acoustic neuroma is only one of many different types of brain tumors (other types are discussed below), but it is among the more common ones. This brain tumor affects 1 in 100,000 people in the United States every year, and in the majority of cases only one ear is affected. A much rarer form of acoustic neuroma, bilateral acoustic neurofibromatosis, is a hereditary condition that affects both ears.

Diagnosing Acoustic Neuroma. Because the early symptoms of acoustic neuroma are very subtle, they may be neglected until the tumor has grown large and is causing more significant symptoms. The early symptoms include a slight hearing loss in the affected ear with or without tinnitus (ringing or buzzing in the ear). Any difference in hearing between the two ears or tinnitus in one ear needs to be fully evaluated. Natural degenerative and aging changes affect both ears equally, and there is no such thing as aging changes in one ear only. Therefore it is important to get a thorough examination and evaluation. Even though an acoustic neuroma is a benign condition, that doesn't mean it can't cause serious harm. If left untreated, it can grow and severely affect hearing and balance, as well as compress the brain stem and other nerves, causing numbness or paralysis of the face, hoarseness, headache, and other symptoms.

To help make a diagnosis, a neurotologist, otorhinolaryngologist, or neurologist will likely conduct an audiogram, the auditory brain stem response test, and the electronystagmography battery of tests, which, in cases of acoustic neuroma, would indicate that something was affecting the eighth cranial nerve. The specialist would probably then order an MRI to confirm the diagnosis.

Treatment. Surgery is the usual treatment for these tumors. Because acoustic neuromas typically grow very slowly, and depending on the patient's age, some doctors suggest that some patients who have very small tumors "watch and wait" and undergo periodic MRI scans to monitor the tumor's progress. As the tumor grows, however, the risk of experiencing worsening balance problems and developing permanent hearing loss increases, and surgery is indicated.

Removal of the tumor will not restore any hearing loss that occurred before the surgery, but balance is nearly always completely restored once the brain learns to compensate, especially when patients take part in vestibular rehabilitation therapy (see chapter 12). If surgery is performed before balance is affected significantly, rehabilitation therapy may or may not be needed, depending on the overall health, age, and needs of the individual patient.

Brian's Story. Brian is a 56-year-old tow truck company owner who came to see me complaining that there was ringing and loss of some hearing in his right ear. He had been experiencing these symptoms for several years and had tried to ignore them. Now he was concerned, however, because he could no longer hear on the phone in his right ear and he was occasionally having some problems with feeling slightly off balance and unsteady on his feet.

Before coming to see me, Brian had gone to his general practitioner, who had found nothing unusual during his examination, and so he referred Brian to me. I ordered a hearing test, which showed hearing loss in the right ear that was worse at higher frequencies. Then I sent Brian for an MRI, which revealed an acoustic neuroma (2.5 centimeters in diameter) that was compressing his eighth cranial nerve. Fortunately it had not yet grown large enough to affect his brain stem.

We discussed his options, and Brian elected to have the tumor removed rather than wait to see how much it grew. Brian recovered quickly without a need for vestibular rehabilitation therapy, and there was no return of his symptoms.

Brian could have chosen to wait and see how much the tumor would grow. His balance problems were subtle, which is common when the brain stem is not involved. If the tumor had been allowed to grow, it could have affected his brain stem and cerebellum; this would have resulted in significant balance problems, headache, and more significant hearing loss. Some tumors also affect the trigeminal nerve (also known as the fifth cranial nerve, it travels from the brain stem and affects the face) and can cause facial numbness.

OTHER BRAIN TUMORS

Other types of brain tumors—and there are about a dozen different kinds—can also cause balance problems. Collectively, the number of brain tumors diagnosed in the United States in 2002 was approximately 186,000, of which 150,000 were metastatic tumors (cancerous tumors that spread to the brain from another location in the body) and about 36,000 were primary (those that originated and stayed in the brain). According to the American Brain Tumor Association, the prevalence of brain tumors in the United States is about 131 of every 100,000 people.

How to Recognize Brain Tumors. For many of these people, the first symptom of a brain tumor is a headache that comes and goes, that does not throb, and that is usually worse in the morning. Other common symptoms include problems with balance, seizures, behavior changes, nausea and vomiting, ringing in the ears, double vision, weakness or paralysis, decreased muscle control, and problems with memory, speech, smell, taste, and concentration.

The symptoms of these various types of brain tumors, like those of acoustic neuromas, often mimic those of other diseases; this can make these tumors difficult to diagnose. Another problem is that symptoms often develop gradually and may be subtle, so a long time may pass between when the symptoms begin and when the tumor is diagnosed.

The location of the tumor determines the symptoms. For example, a tumor on the brain stem causes hearing loss, balance problems, double vision, and a reduction in facial sensation. However, a tumor that develops between the brain stem and cerebellum may cause dizziness, tremors, staggering, headache, nausea, and vomiting.

Diagnosis and Treatment. Diagnosis of brain tumors is similar to that of an acoustic neuroma, with an MRI often being the definitive test, as very few brain tumors escape this imaging technique. Treatment depends on the type of tumor. A benign tumor typically grows very slowly and rarely spreads. However, surgical removal is usually recommended, especially if the tumor is located in an area of the brain involved with vital functions, such as breathing and movement. Once the tumor is removed, no additional treatment is usually required.

Malignant brain tumors, also called brain cancer, grow rapidly, spread, and are life threatening. They may require immediate removal, and their removal may be followed up with chemotherapy (anticancer drugs) and/or radiation to prevent recurrence.

EPILEPSY

Epilepsy is a brain disorder in which clusters of nerve cells send abnormal electric signals that can result in unusual sensations, behaviors, emotions, and loss of consciousness. Most people equate epilepsy with seizures and no other symptoms, because people with epilepsy often experience muscle spasms, convulsions, repeated hand rubbing and lip smacking, and other unusual movements. Yet one of the most common types of epilepsy, called temporal lobe epilepsy, is usually characterized by other symptoms, including dizziness, lightheadedness, faintness, shortness of breath, palpitations, and sweating.

Approximately 2 million Americans have active epilepsy,

which means they have been treated with drugs to control their seizures for at least five years. Epilepsy affects men more often than women. Each year, about 125,000 new cases of epilepsy occur, and about 30 percent of them appear among children, especially during the first year of life. New cases also are common among the elderly.

If you have experienced symptoms of epilepsy, be sure to tell your doctor about them, including any unusual sensations, movements, or behaviors. Epilepsy is typically diagnosed once the doctor gets a thorough medical history, completes a neurological examination, and gets the results of an electroencephalogram (EEG), a procedure that measures the electric activity of your brain via electrodes that are placed on your head. Occasionally a CT or MRI is also ordered to see if there are any tumors, cysts, signs of stroke, or other brain abnormalities that could be causing the seizures.

How to Treat Epilepsy. For about 75 percent of the 2 million people who have epilepsy, a single medication—one of many anticonvulsants on the market—can control their seizures. For about 600,000 people, however, the medications either do not work or cause debilitating side effects. These individuals may elect to undergo a surgical procedure that removes the part of the brain from which the abnormal electric activity originates. Surgery isn't an option if there is more than one such area in the brain or if the area can't be removed because it is involved in vital bodily functions.

HEAD TRAUMA

You've already seen how trauma to the head or ear can cause specific types of vestibular disorders (e.g., benign paroxysmal positional vertigo and perilymphatic fistula), but such events can also cause nonspecific damage to your vestibular system. If you experience any dizziness, vertigo, imbalance, vision problems, hearing loss, or ringing in your ears after suffering a blow to the head or experiencing any type of head or neck injury, such as whiplash or a sports injury, you should see your doctor immediately.

According to the National Head Injury Foundation, about 2 million new cases of traumatic brain injury occur each year. Dizziness, giddiness, and periodic lightheadedness affect up to 78 percent of the people who experience a head injury, even a mild one, and these symptoms can last for months, even years, after the event.

Sometimes symptoms don't appear for days, weeks, or months after the injury has occurred, and this time delay causes many people not to link the present symptoms with a head injury they suffered months previously. All they know is that they turned their head quickly and suddenly they were dizzy, for no apparent reason. Thus, always report any past head injuries to your doctor.

Cervical Vertigo. Neck injuries, including whiplash injuries that may or may not involve head trauma, also can be associated with balance problems. A syndrome known as cervical vertigo, characterized by disequilibrium, vertigo, and limited neck mobility, can occur in people who have had a neck injury. It is believed that a misalignment of the cervical joints in the neck alter the signals that travel from the proprioceptive system (skin, joints, and muscles) to the vestibular system, resulting in balance problems. Muscle spasms in the neck are also associated with dizziness. People with cervical vertigo often respond to chiropractic and physical therapy (see chapter 15).

Margaret's Story. About six months before she finally came to my office, Margaret, a 36-year-old sales representative, had been a passenger in a car that had been struck on the driver's side. She suffered a blow to the right side of her head on the passenger-side window but she didn't lose consciousness, and a CT scan did not show a concussion. For several months she went for weekly chiropractic treatments for relief of neck pain, frequent headaches, dizziness, and problems with balance, which she noticed especially when she was in poorly lit environments. While the pain and headaches eventually disappeared, the dizziness and difficulty maintaining her balance did not.

In addition to the symptoms already mentioned, Margaret noted that she was having some trouble hearing in her right ear. We performed caloric testing and rotary chair testing, which showed a weak response in her right ear. An audiogram revealed sensorineural hearing loss in her right ear and normal hearing in her left. Her Dix-Hallpike maneuvers were negative, and she had no vision or sensory problems.

On the basis of her history, physical and neurologic examinations, and other findings, we eliminated other possible diagnoses, including benign positional vertigo, perilymphatic fistula, and brain stem concussion, and diagnosed her with labyrinthine concussion—a concussion of the labyrinth. Her treatment consisted of vestibular rehabilitation therapy (see chapter 12) and a vestibular suppressant, meclizine, which she used as needed (see appendix C). After six months, she was using the meclizine only once or twice a month.

MIGRAINE

Migraine is a common disorder in which there is throbbing pain, most often on one side of the head only, that can be accompanied by nausea, vomiting, sensitivity to sound and light, dizziness, vertigo, and imbalance. More than 20 million people in the United States suffer from migraine, and women are four times more likely to experience the attacks than are men. Migraine attacks can recur every few days, or weeks, months, or years may pass between episodes.

Types of Migraine. The International Headache Society classifies migraine into the following categories:

- Migraine with aura. An aura is a set of symptoms (flashes of light, tingling, vertigo, numbness, and noise) that occur before the head pain begins and lasts about 5 to 20 minutes. Nearly 20 percent of the people who suffer with migraine experience this type, although they do not necessarily have an aura before every migraine.
- Migraine without aura. This is the most common type of migraine and affects about 80 percent of migraine sufferers.

In these two types of migraine, the headache usually builds slowly and can last from several hours to more than a day. Physical activity and light make the pain worse; this is why most people prefer to lie quietly in a dark room until the symptoms pass. Vertigo can occur before, during, or after the head pain.

- Basilar migraine. This is a subtype of migraine with aura and is characterized by vertigo, nausea and vomiting, loss of coordination, ringing in the ears, overall weakness, speech difficulties, and decreased hearing. The vertigo typically lasts 5 to 60 minutes. Some people experience only a moderate headache, or none at all, along with these symptoms and may not tell their doctor about it because they are more concerned about the aura and other symptoms.

This was the case with Michael, a 38-year-old real estate broker who had a strong family and personal history of migraine. When Michael came to my office, he reported episodes of sudden vertigo attacks with nausea and vomiting, without headache, ringing in his ears, hearing problems, or a feeling of fullness in his ears. I conducted a thorough physical examination, as well as a neurological examination and balance and electronystagmography testing. All results were normal. I made a diagnosis of basilar migraine based on the unexplained symptoms without head pain and his strong personal and family history of migraine.

The main treatment for basilar migraine is medications (e.g., antihistamines, antiemetics, and sedatives) to help relieve vertigo and the associated symptoms. People who experience frequent basilar migraines can get some relief by taking beta blockers, a common antimigraine medication (see "Migraine Medications" below).

• Migraine equivalents. These are disorders in which people experience episodes of vertigo, hearing loss, and ringing in the ears but only occasionally or never develop head pain. Migraine equivalents are not common; however, they deserve mention because it can be difficult to differentiate them from cases of Ménière's disease, and treatment of these two conditions differs. One of the more common types of migraine equivalents is benign paroxysmal vertigo of childhood, which is discussed in chapter 4.

Causes and Triggers. Migraine triggers can be as varied as stress, certain foods (especially those that contain nitrates or monosodium glutamate), lack of sleep, hypoglycemia (low blood sugar levels), smoking, use of oral contraceptives, pregnancy, anxiety, fluctuating estrogen levels, and flashing lights. The actual cause of migraine is not completely understood. The pain is believed to be the result of the dilatation, inflammation, or spasm of blood vessels in the brain. The aura may be caused by temporary dysfunction of nerve cells. Dizziness and vertigo may be caused by a temporary reduction of blood flow to the inner ear.

How to Prevent and Treat Migraine. Prevention of migraine can take several forms. The ones that work best for you will depend on what triggers your attacks and their frequency. Here are some guidelines for prevention:

• Eliminate foods and additives that can trigger migraine, such as chocolate, nuts, monosodium glutamate, and foods that contain the chemical tyramine—aged cheeses, pickled herring, and red wine.
• Engage in stress management techniques, including biofeedback, hypnosis, meditation, and yoga.

- Get adequate sleep every night.
- Avoid caffeine and nicotine.
- Take part in daily aerobic exercise for at least 30 minutes.
- Avoid hypoglycemia (low blood sugar levels) by eating something at least every eight hours.
- Take medications designed to abort an impending migraine attack, such as sumatriptan (Imitrex) or zolmitriptan (Zomig). These have about a 70 percent success rate in preventing a migraine attack if they are taken immediately at the first sign of an aura or head pain.
- If migraines occur frequently or if drugs to abort an attack aren't very effective, you may choose to take daily preventive medication, such as tricyclic antidepressants, beta-blockers, or calcium channel blockers (see below).

Migraine Medications. Once a migraine attack occurs, many people find that lying in a dark room, taking medications that help improve blood flow (e.g., beta-blockers and calcium channel blockers) and manage nausea and vomiting (e.g., antiemetics), and sleeping are the most effective strategies. Helpful medications include the following. Talk to your doctor about which drugs are best for you.

- Antimigraine medications (e.g., sumatriptan [Imitrex] and zolmitriptan [Zomig]) may prevent a migraine if taken at the first indication of an attack. These drugs are available as tablets, injections (self-administered; sumatriptan), and nasal sprays (sumatriptan). Side effects include drowsiness or dizziness, and burning, pain, or redness at the injection site (sumatriptan). You should not use these drugs if you have angina pectoris, uncontrolled high blood pressure, or a history of a heart condition.
- Tricyclic antidepressants (e.g., amitriptyline [Elavil], desipramine [Norpramin], doxepin [Sinequan], and nortriptyline [Pamelor]) have proved effective in controlling ver-

tigo in patients with migraine. Side effects include dry mouth, dry eyes, constipation, and reduced urinary flow.

- Antiemetics (e.g., prochlorperazine [Compazine] and metoclopramide [Maxolon, Octamide, and Reglan) are used specifically to stop nausea and vomiting. Side effects can include blurry vision, drowsiness, dizziness, lightheadedness, weight gain, dry mouth, and constipation.
- Beta-blockers (e.g., atenolol [Tenormin], metaprolol [Lopressor], propranolol [Inderal], nadolol [Corgard], and timolol [Blocadren]) help prevent the blood vessels from expanding. Side effects can include drowsiness; cold hands and feet; dry mouth, eyes, and skin; and dizziness.
- Calcium channel blockers (e.g., nifedipine [Adalat], nimodipine [Nimotop], and verapamil [Calan]) dilate the small blood vessels of the inner ear, to improve blood flow. Unfortunately, side effects of these drugs can include dizziness, lightheadedness, flushing, weakness, and diarrhea, although these effects are usually mild.

MULTIPLE SCLEROSIS

Multiple sclerosis is a disease of the central nervous system in which the myelin—a material that covers nerve cells—is destroyed or damaged, a process called demyelination. This causes the signals that normally pass among nerve cells to be interrupted. Depending on the areas of the body in which demyelination occurs, people with multiple sclerosis can experience dizziness, balance problems, and vertigo. In fact, up to 50 percent of the people with multiple sclerosis experience vertigo as part of their illness, and in 5 percent of the people, vertigo is the initial symptom of the disease.

Experts are not certain why demyelination occurs, but research indicates that multiple sclerosis is an autoimmune disease. That means, for reasons unknown, the body's immune system turns against itself and damages healthy cells.

Approximately 350,000 people in the United States have been diagnosed with multiple sclerosis, but the number may be greater because of the difficulty in identifying the disease. In about 90 percent of the people diagnosed, the symptoms first appear between the ages of 20 and 40, and women are twice as likely to get the disease as men.

How to Recognize Multiple Sclerosis. For many people, the first symptoms include sudden blurriness or lost vision in one eye (in about 20 percent of patients) or numbness in the arms or legs (up to 55 percent of patients). Both of these symptoms may last for a few weeks and then improve. One or both of these symptoms can have a significant effect on balance and gait. The extent of nerve damage in the eyes, spinal cord, and nervous system determines the extent and seriousness of balance problems.

In addition to the symptoms already mentioned, people with multiple sclerosis can also experience pain, muscle weakness, hearing loss, slurred speech, loss of bladder and bowel function, gastrointestinal problems, headache, and other symptoms. Individuals vary greatly in how the disease affects them. For some, one or two symptoms appear and remain mild for months or years before they get any worse. During that time a new symptom may or may not appear. Other people get a few moderate or severe symptoms from the start and then acquire new ones as time passes. Regardless of the severity of symptoms, it appears that all people with multiple sclerosis experience a continual loss of brain tissue.

Subsequent attacks of the same initial symptoms or different ones may occur within weeks, months, or even years. All of this unpredictability makes it difficult to diagnose multiple sclerosis, especially when most people don't keep track of their various symptoms, how and when they occurred and for how long they lasted. It helps to keep a diary of symptoms so you can best help your health-care provider make an accurate diagnosis.

Diagnosis. Diagnosis of multiple sclerosis can be difficult, especially in its early stages when identifying nerve abnormalities is not always clear. After your doctor takes your medical history, a neurological exam will be done to test your reflexes, limb strength, sensation, and coordination. An eye exam will determine whether there has been any damage to your optic nerve. Electronystagmography to detect nystagmus and auditory and visual evoked responses can be especially helpful in diagnosing multiple sclerosis. Two types of nystagmus are often seen in multiple sclerosis but are unusual in other diseases.

An MRI is very sensitive in revealing areas of the brain where demyelination has occurred, although this approach isn't helpful in about 25 percent of the people who are in the early stages of the disease. A sample of cerebrospinal fluid taken from the spine can be an accurate indication of multiple sclerosis, because about 90 percent of the people with the disease have a characteristic called oligoclonal bands in their fluid.

How to Treat Multiple Sclerosis. So far there are no effective treatments for the underlying cause of multiple sclerosis. Treatment typically consists of medications to relieve the various symptoms, especially pain, numbness and tingling, muscle weakness, and bladder and bowel problems. Unfortunately, many of the drugs prescribed for these symptoms (e.g., tricyclic antidepressants, anticonvulsants, and sedatives) can cause dizziness as well as other side effects (see chapter 9 for information on these drugs). Another class of drugs used to treat some multiple sclerosis patients is beta-interferons, which are not associated with dizziness but do cause a wide range of other side effects.

PARKINSON'S DISEASE

Parkinson's disease typically affects older adults, but it was brought into the spotlight near the turn of the millennium when a highly popular young actor, Michael J. Fox, was struck by the disorder at the age of 29. Parkinson's disease is a movement disorder; in fact, one of its most common symptoms is poor balance, especially when individuals try to move suddenly. This can result in falls, which it does in more than 35 percent of people who have an advanced form of the disease.

Parkinson's disease is characterized by a severe deficiency of a chemical substance in the brain called dopamine. Dopamine allows people to move smoothly and normally; thus a shortage of this chemical results in symptoms that can make the lives of those with Parkinson's disease an everyday challenge.

How to Recognize Parkinson's Disease. In addition to poor balance, other common symptoms of Parkinson's disease include the following:

- Tremors, which may be worse on one side of the body. Usually affect the legs and arms as well as the head, neck, and face. Up to 25 percent of patients experience mild or no tremors at all.
- Rigidity, or stiffness of the muscles. Can be relieved with anti-Parkinson's medications, but these drugs also have a tendency to produce dizziness and postural hypotension in some people (see chapter 9).
- Difficulty walking that is the result of the shuffling steps, reduced or nonexistent arm swing, problems when turning, and spontaneous episodes of being unable to take a step (called "freezing spells") that are characteristic of Parkinson's disease.
- Slow movements, also known as bradykinesia. Individuals who have Parkinson's often experience a delay when initiating a movement, such as taking a step or raising their arm, because there is a slowdown in the transmission of signals by the brain to the targeted body part.
- Other symptoms which may include dizziness, stooped posture, sleep problems, depression, constipation, and difficulties with speech, breathing, and swallowing.

How to Treat Parkinson's Disease. The mainstay of treatment of Parkinson's disease is a combination of two drugs: levodopa and carbidopa. Why two? Levodopa is converted into dopamine, which the brain needs, but much of it is metabolized before it even gets to the brain. That's where carbidopa comes in. This drug increases the amount of levodopa that reaches the brain. The result of this combination drug (Sinemet) is that rigidity, bradykinesia, and tremors are controlled; however, balance problems are not managed as well by these drugs. Side effects include gastrointestinal distress and hypotension.

Other drugs can also be used along with levodopa. Selegiline (Carbex) helps increase the amount of dopamine in the brain, but it also can cause dizziness, nausea, confusion, dry mouth, and hallucinations. A new class of drugs called COMT (catechol-O-methyl transferase) inhibitors, when taken with levodopa, boost the amount of levodopa that enters the brain. The two drugs currently available, Entacapone (Comtan) and tolcapone (Tasmar), can cause side effects that include visual hallucinations, nausea, sleep problems, vivid dreams, daytime drowsiness, headache, and problems with voluntary movement.

INFECTIONS OF THE CENTRAL NERVOUS SYSTEM

Infections of the central nervous system can cause dizziness, vertigo, and/or disequilibrium. In some cases, dizziness is the only symptom of the infection that individuals notice initially. These infections are common enough that doctors consider them when making a diagnosis, and so you should be aware of them and the symptoms they can cause.

Syphilis. Syphilis is caused by a bacterium, *Treponema pallidum*, typically spread via sexual contact, although it can also be passed from an infected mother to her unborn child. People who have syphilis often remain without symptoms (asymptomatic) for years, and thus often don't seek treatment because they don't know something is wrong. When the disease reaches the central nervous system, which can take from one to three years after the initial infection, dizziness is common and can be the initial symptom.

If you are experiencing dizziness that you and your health-care practitioner cannot explain, he or she may order a blood test to determine if syphilis is the cause. More than 104 people per day are diagnosed with syphilis, and most of them are between the ages of 20 and 39. Fortunately, treatment with penicillin or other antibiotics is usually effective and can eliminate the disease and, along with it, the dizziness.

If, however, syphilis goes untreated for ten years or more, a deterioration of the spinal cord can occur, causing permanent disequilibrium. Sometimes the syphilis reaches the labyrinth and causes symptoms of Ménière's disease, including vertigo, ringing in the ears, and fullness in the ears.

Lyme Disease. Receive just one bite from a deer tick that is carrying the bacterium *Borrelia burgdorferi,* and you could have Lyme disease. A characteristic telltale sign of Lyme disease is a bull's eye rash where the tick bit, but some people miss seeing the tick bite or do not develop the rash. If Lyme disease goes unnoticed, the disease can progress, and symptoms such as dizziness, fever, joint aches, malaise, fatigue, and headache develop.

Treatment of Lyme disease typically involves taking antibiotics for three to four weeks if the disease is caught in the early stages. More-prolonged antibiotic therapy is needed if you don't detect the disease until its later stages.

You're at risk of contracting Lyme disease if you live in a state that has a significant tick population. These include states in the northeast, mid-Atlantic, and upper-north-central part of the United States. More than 16,000 people get the disease per year.

Meningitis. Meningitis is an infectious condition that can be caused by a virus, bacterium, or fungus, although most cases are viral or bacterial. The infection affects the meninges (membranes) that cover the brain and spinal cord. Telltale symptoms of all forms of the disease include dizziness, fever, headache, confusion, drowsiness, and a stiff neck.

One of the lingering effects of bacterial meningitis is disequilibrium. Even after the infection has been resolved, residual damage from the infection, which can include swelling anywhere in the vestibular system, invasion of the bacteria into the labyrinth resulting in labyrinthitis (see chapter 4), or injury to the cerebellum, can result in balance problems that last for months. Other aftereffects include giddiness, recurring headache, difficulty concentrating, short-term memory loss, depression, aggressive behavior, deafness, ringing in the ears, and joint stiffness, among others. Worldwide, 1.2 million people develop bacterial meningitis annually, and 135,000 die of it. One in seven survivors lives with severe handicaps as a result of the disease.

Viral meningitis is usually less serious. Fortunately, it typically resolves without treatment, as antibiotics are ineffective against this form of the disease.

Cardiovascular System Disorders

The cardiovascular system—the heart and all the various types of blood vessels—is responsible for pumping blood, oxygen, and nutrients throughout the body. When that system is compromised in any way and the heart beats too fast, too slow, irregularly, or not at all or when one or more blood vessels is partly or completely blocked, lightheadedness, dizziness, or disequilibrium can result. Usually a balance or dizziness problem is just one of many symptoms that are part of a cardiovascular system disorder.

A brief cardiovascular examination is a routine part of a physical examination (see chapter 3). However, if you have a history of heart problems or have one or more risk factors for cardiovascular disease or if your doctor detects an abnormality in your heart during this examination, you may be referred to a cardiologist for further evaluation. Those risk factors include a family history of cardiovascular disease, high total blood cholesterol levels (elevated LDL [low-density lipoprotein] and too-low HDL [high-density lipoprotein] levels), high lipid (fat) levels in the blood, obesity, diabetes, smoking, and physical inactivity.

Here are some of the cardiovascular conditions that often have lightheadedness, dizziness, and/or disequilibrium associated with them.

ARRYTHMIAS

Arrythmias are episodes of irregular, too fast, or too slow heart beat frequently brought on by sudden emotional stress or physical pain. Although a routine electrocardiogram (EKG) can identify most types of serious heart disease, you should undergo EKG monitoring if you are experiencing intermittent arrhythmias and near-dizziness. Unlike a routine EKG, which shows your heart's performance at one point in time, monitoring allows your doctor to track the abnormalities in your rhythm over a 24-hour period (or longer). This monitoring, called Holter monitoring, involves wearing a lightweight portable device that has electrodes that are attached to your chest and record your heartbeat.

Samuel's Story. Samuel, a 58-year-old plumber, was sitting by the pool, watching his grandchildren play when he suddenly felt lightheaded and experienced palpitations. The episode lasted for about a minute, so he blamed it on being in the sun too long. Later that night, however, he was still feeling lightheaded, even after making sure he had taken in enough fluids, so his wife insisted he see his doctor as soon as possible.

When Samuel's doctor asked him about the episode, he admitted that he had had another one a week earlier, but had not told his wife. Samuel's doctor checked his heart with a stethoscope and took his blood pressure, and then referred him to a cardiologist. The cardiologist performed an EKG and monitored his heart with Holter monitoring for 24 hours. He diagnosed Samuel with atrial fibrillation, a condition in which the upper chambers of the heart (atria) contract rapidly, causing episodes of palpitations, lightheadedness, chest discomfort, shortness of breath, or fainting. Samuel was prescribed medication (diltiazem) to help regulate his arrhythmias and was told to switch to a low-fat diet. If his case had been more severe, his cardiologist may have suggested a pacemaker.

ORTHOSTATIC HYPOTENSION

If you have ever experienced lightheadedness, giddiness, a swimming sensation in your head, or a feeling that you were going to faint after you've stood up from a seated or lying position, you've experienced orthostatic hypotension. For many people, these fleeting spells of dizziness occur occasionally and are inconsequential. For others, however, the symptoms recur daily. Especially among the elderly, orthostatic hypotension is a major cause of disequilibrium, which creates an increased risk of falls and fractures.

What Causes Orthostatic Hypotension? When you stand from a seated or lying position, it takes your body approximately 60 seconds to adjust to the change in position. During that time, your heart rate may increase by 10 to 15 beats per minute, and you may have an increase in blood pressure as well. By the time the minute is up, your body has stabilized and your heart rate and blood pressure have returned to normal.

Other situations that can lead to orthostatic hypotension include the following:

- When there is too little blood volume, which can occur if you have anemia, if you are dehydrated, or if you are undergoing dialysis

- If you are taking certain medications, such as those taken to treat high blood pressure, heart disease, or depression, as they can weaken the blood vessels' ability to constrict, and so cause blood pressure to fall
- When blood vessels dilate, which can occur when you are taking a hot shower, have a fever, are in a hot environment
- After eating, when more blood is delegated to the digestive process than to the brain and other areas of the body
- If there is a disorder in the part of the nervous system that helps regulate blood pressure (the autonomic nervous system)
- If you have benign paroxysmal positional vertigo (discussed in chapter 4)
- If you have a condition called postural orthostatic tachycardia (POTS) syndrome, in which the pulse rate increases by 30 beats or more per minute within ten minutes of standing from a lying position

Diagnosing Orthostatic Hypotension. To test for orthostatic hypotension, your doctor will take your blood pressure, first while you are lying down and then while you are standing. Orthostatic hypotension is defined as a decline of at least 20 millimeters of mercury in your systolic blood pressure (the top number in a blood pressure reading; e.g., 120 in a reading of 120/80) along with an increase in pulse rate. To uncover its cause, your doctor should take a thorough history and then, on the basis of that information, he or she may order blood tests (to look for anemia), a glucose tolerance test (for diabetes), an EKG (for heart irregularities), a test for electrolyte levels (for dehydration), or any number of other tests. In some difficult to diagnose cases, a tilt-table test may be necessary to clinch the diagnosis. During this test the heart rate and blood pressure are monitored while the table is tilted and to gauge their response to certain medications.

Treatment. Orthostatic hypotension is typically treated by stopping the offending medication, correcting or managing the underlying medical condition (e.g., anemia or diabetes), or, if the cause is related to the autonomic nervous system, increasing the amount of salt in the diet to increase blood volume. Fluorocortisone, a drug that helps raise blood volume by assisting the body in retaining salt, can be used in serious cases. Once you begin the correct treatment, your dizziness should eventually cease.

STRUCTURAL HEART DISEASE

Structural heart disease refers to conditions in which there are physical abnormalities in the heart that can lead to heart failure and reduced blood flow to the brain, thus causing lightheadedness and dizziness. The most common disorders include the following:

• Cardiomyopathy is a disease of the heart muscle in which either the heart enlarges and becomes weak (the most common form of cardiomyopathy) or the heart muscle thickens but continues to beat strongly. Lightheadedness, dizziness, and fainting can be symptoms of either form, but more often of the former. Other symptoms include shortness of breath, chest pain, palpitations, high blood pressure, fatigue, reduced concentration, and swollen ankles, legs, or other parts of the body. Treatment typically includes various heart medications (e.g., calcium channel blockers, ACE inhibitors, and diuretics), dietary changes (low-fat, high-fiber diet), and stress management.

• Myocardial infarction, better known as a heart attack, occurs when there is a severe or prolonged decrease in oxygen to the heart, caused by blockage in an artery. The blockage is usually the result of atherosclerosis, the buildup of plaque in the blood vessels. A myocardial infarction causes part of the heart muscle to die. In addition to dizziness or fainting, other symptoms of a myocardial infarction include unexplained weakness or fatigue, rapid or irregular pulse, nausea or vomiting, shortness of breath, and cool, clammy skin and/or paleness.

- Valvular disease is characterized by a malfunction or abnormality of one or more of the four valves in the heart. Dizziness is a symptom of the two most common types of valvular diseases: mitral valve prolapse and regurgitation and aortic valve stenosis.

  - In mitral valve prolapse, the valve that links the upper and lower chambers on the left side of the heart malfunctions and balloons out (prolapses). About 5 percent of the population has this disorder. Typical symptoms include dizziness, vertigo, migraines, balance problems, insomnia, hyperventilation, heart palpitations, panic attacks, difficulty concentrating, cold sweats, cold hands and feet, and bowel problems, as well as a slightly increased risk of infection of the heart. If there are few or no symptoms, treatment may include stress management, exercise, and attention to diet (avoiding caffeine, alcohol, and sugar). Antiarrhythmic drugs may be needed if irregular heart rhythms are present, or propranolol (Inderal, a beta-blocker) may be given for palpitations. More serious cases may require surgical repair or replacement of the valve.

  - In aortic valve stenosis, the aortic valve is scarred and reduces the outflow of the pumping heart, causing the heart to pump harder. The reduced blood flow causes dizziness, lightheadedness, shortness of breath, fainting, swollen ankles, and chest pain. If symptoms are mild, the disease usually can be treated with diuretics. In more serious cases, the valve usually needs to be replaced with an artificial one because the aortic valve typically cannot be repaired. Aortic valve stenosis affects about 5 out of every 10,000 (0.05%) people.

TRANSIENT ISCHEMIC ATTACKS

A transient ischemic attack (TIA, or little stroke) occurs when there is a temporary reduction of blood flow (ischemia) to a portion of the brain. Characteristic symptoms of a TIA include vertigo, problems with balance and coordination, tingling or numbness (usually on one side of the body), blurry vision, and slurred speech.

The interruption in the blood supply may be caused by plaque that has accumulated on the walls of the arteries that supply the brain, which restricts blood flow, or by clots that travel from another location in the body and then block small arteries. Blockages that last for more than a few minutes usually cause a more serious condition—stroke (see below).

Sylvia's Story. Symptoms of a TIA vary, depending on the area of the brain that is affected. Sylvia, a 57-year-old fashion designer, was busy at her drawing board one Monday morning when she suddenly experienced double vision and had difficulty holding the pencil in her right hand. When she tried to stand, the room began to spin, and she fell to the floor. Fortunately, her husband was in the other room and came to her aid. After a few minutes, Sylvia felt much better and was ready to dismiss the episode, but her husband insisted she see a doctor. She refused, arguing that she didn't have high blood pressure and she had no history of diabetes, heart disease, or smoking, but her husband was persistent. Reluctantly, she made an appointment for Wednesday morning.

Sylvia was wise to listen to her husband, although she would have been smarter if she had gone to the emergency room at the time. A TIA is a warning that something is amiss within the cerebrovascular system (blood supply to the brain), and the warning should be taken seriously. In fact, about one-third of people who have a TIA have a stroke in the future, another third go on to have one or more TIAs, and the other third are fortunate in not having another episode. It doesn't pay to gamble that you'll be among that final third when the stakes are this high.

One reason the stakes are high is that even when blood flow is reduced for just a few seconds, brain cells in the affected area die, producing permanent damage. The level of damage may be slight after the first TIA or it may be significant and include problems with loss of vision, slurred speech, loss of balance, reduced sensation in parts of the body, and concentration difficulties. Sylvia is at increased risk because she is older than 50, the age at which the incidence of TIAs rises dramatically. She does not fall into the other high-risk categories, however: TIAs are also more common among men and blacks.

Treatment. Because TIAs are a warning of possible future events, the goal of treatment is to prevent stroke by improving the blood supply to the brain. Also, anyone who has a condition that contributes to the development of TIAs or stroke, such as diabetes, heart disease, high blood pressure, high cholesterol, or a blood disorder, needs to have that condition identified and treated as well. Lifestyle changes, such as stopping smoking, eating a low-fat, low-salt diet, and getting sufficient exercise, also are an essential part of treatment.

In Sylvia's case, her medical history and physical examination didn't show anything significant to explain why she had experienced a TIA. However, this finding was not a license for her to disregard the incident. To help ensure her future would be TIA- and stroke-free, her doctor encouraged her to adopt a healthier diet (low-fat, low-salt, more fruits and vegetables), to lose 20 pounds, and to take an aspirin every other day to reduce the tendency of the blood to clot and thus improve blood flow to the brain.

STROKE

Sudden dizziness, loss of coordination or balance, or difficulty walking—this group of symptoms is one of the five classic warning signs of a stroke. A stroke, also known as a cerebrovascular incident or a "brain attack," occurs when the blood supply to the brain is interrupted for a few minutes or more, resulting in permanent damage to and death of brain cells in the affected areas. This differs from a TIA, in which blood flow stops for only a few seconds.

According to the American Stroke Association, a stroke occurs every 53 seconds in the United States. Strokes affect 600,000 people per year, of whom 160,000 will die, making stroke the number three cause of death in the United States. Overall, two-thirds of the strokes happen to people older than 65.

Warning Signs. There are five common warning signs of an impending stroke, and the occurrence of any one is reason to call 911 immediately. We've already mentioned one of the warning signs—a TIA. The other four are:

- Sudden weakness or numbness of the face, leg, or arm, especially on one side of the body
- Sudden difficulty speaking or understanding, or sudden confusion
- Sudden difficulty seeing in one or both eyes
- Sudden severe headache that has no apparent cause

Risk Factors. Among the many risk factors for stroke, the most important (and those you can control) are high blood pressure, smoking, diabetes, heart disease, and a history of TIAs. In fact, your risk of having a stroke increases 10 times if you have had one or more TIAs. People with heart disease have more than twice the risk of having a stroke than those without heart problems.

Treatment. Stroke can be treated, and with some success, if you seek emergency medical assistance. The type of medical treatment depends on the type of stroke. The most common kind of stroke (which affects more than 50 percent of the people who suffer a stroke) is an ischemic, or thrombotic, stroke in which there is a clot blocking blood flow. For this condition, doctors can prescribe "clot-busting" medications, such as t-Pa, or blood-thinning drugs, such as warfarin. Other options are medical procedures such as angioplasty, in which doctors unclog fatty buildup in the blocked artery by inserting a balloon catheter into the artery to widen it, or carotid endarterectomy, in which the blockage is surgically removed.

In addition to medical treatment, rehabilitation is a critical part of recovery from a stroke. If you've had a stroke and have difficulties with balance or coordination, vestibular rehabilitation therapy can be very effective in helping you regain some or even most of your independence, strength, and functioning, depending on the severity of the damage to your nervous system.

VERTEBROBASILAR INSUFFICIENCY

If you have a temporary blockage of the arteries in the back of the neck that supply the brain with blood, you may experience vertigo that lasts several minutes and be accompanied by nausea and vomiting. In about 29 percent of cases, visual problems (blurry or double vision) also occur, while unsteadiness, extreme weakness, confusion, headache, and hearing loss occur in less than 10 percent of the people affected.

Such episodes are attributed to vertebrobasilar insufficiency, which gets its name from the fact that the impaired blood flow affects the vertebral or basilar arteries. The most common cause is atherosclerosis (hardening of these same arteries), but it may also be caused by diabetes, polycythemia (see chapter 7), arteritis (inflammation of the arteries), and conditions in which the blood clots too easily (hypercoagulation).

Attacks of vertigo associated with vertebrobasilar insufficiency can occur simply by turning your neck farther than usual, which causes the arteries to twist and become more narrow momentarily. For example, have you ever suddenly turned your head in the car to yell at your kids in the backseat, or reached behind you from the front seat of the car to get something off the backseat? The rapid twist of your head can cause a temporary disruption in blood flow, which can be enough to cause the attack, especially in older people who have a more narrow vertebral or spinal column.

To treat vertebrobasilar insufficiency, you must identify the cause and then manage that condition. Treatment often includes taking blood-thinning drugs (e.g., aspirin).

Bottom Line

Millions of people live with cardiovascular or central nervous system disorders. For some individuals, a feeling of lightheadedness, dizziness, spinning, or unsteadiness on their feet may be their first clue that something is wrong, and it may be the symptom that prompts them to go to their doctor. After a thorough examination, history taking, and appropriate testing, an underlying cardiovascular or central nervous system disorder may be identified.

For other individuals, this symptom is just one or more among many others they experience as part of their disease. In either situation, it is necessary to treat the underlying condition in order to effectively deal with the dizziness. In cases where it is appropriate, doctors may recommend balance rehabilitation therapy to complement other treatments they have prescribed.

7

Systemic Disorders

Sometimes there are problems in the body—rather than in the inner ear or brain—that can cause dizziness, vertigo, and/or disequilibrium and their associated symptoms. These problems are referred to as systemic disorders, because they affect the body system as a whole. Not everyone agrees as to which disorders should be included in this category, and in fact, a few rightfully belong in more than one group. So, if you don't see a specific condition in this chapter, feel free to check out chapters 8 and 9, as you may find it there.

That being said, in this chapter we look at allergies, anemia, chronic fatigue immune deficiency syndrome, diabetes, poly-cythemia, rheumatoid arthritis, systemic lupus erythematosus, and thyroid disorders. It's important for you to understand that treatment of these underlying medical conditions is generally necessary in order to get relief from dizziness and associated symptoms.

Allergies

When spring rolls around, do you spend a lot of time sneezing, rubbing itchy eyes, and feeling slightly off-balance? When you eat certain foods, do you get dizzy spells, a headache, or ringing in your ears? Nasal and food allergies can cause a wide variety of symptoms that many people don't recognize as being associated with allergic reactions. Besides a runny nose, watery eyes, and an itchy mouth, nasal (airborne) allergens (substances that cause an allergic reaction) can also trigger dizziness, decreased hearing, increased ear pressure, and vertigo.

WHAT ARE ALLERGIES?

An allergic response is a reaction by the immune system to an irritant, or allergen. An allergen can be any substance that you inhale, ingest, or touch that causes such a reaction. Common allergens include pollen, mold spores, dust, and pet dander (inhaled); peanuts, wheat, dairy products, and monosodium glutamate (ingested); and latex (contact). Dizziness and balance problems are associated with inhaled and ingested allergens.

ALLERGIES AND BALANCE

During an allergy attack, the body releases a number of chemicals, including histamine, serotonin, and many others, that cause inflammation, and that can include inflammation of the inner ear. Nasal allergies can cause the Eustachian tube (the tube between the space in the middle ear to the back of the nose; it helps equalize pressure between the middle ear and the outside) to malfunction, which can cause dizziness, vertigo, ringing in the ears, and decreased hearing.

If you have an inner ear disorder or injury as well as allergies, you can expect the symptoms of your ailment to be aggravated during allergy season. This double trouble can occur because the

Eustachian tube becomes congested, which increases the pressure in the middle and inner ears, or because a direct inflammatory reaction within the inner ear is triggered by the allergen (serous labyrinthitis).

DIAGNOSIS

Your health-care provider can conduct tests to determine which allergens are responsible for your allergic responses. One such test is the immunoglobulin radioallergosorbent test, or Ig RAST, which uses a blood sample to measure the blood antibodies to food antigens. If your test shows high levels of antibodies, it means your body is attacking the proteins of a specific food or inhaled substance in your system.

Another type of test is provocation skin testing, which is very accurate for both airborne and food allergies and sensitivities. Your doctor will inject a minute amount of the suspected allergens under your skin and wait to see if a reddened spot appears at any of the sites. If spots appear, it means you are allergic or sensitive to the substances tested.

HOW TO TREAT ALLERGIES

The best "treatment" for allergies is prevention: simply avoid the allergen. This is not always possible, however, and so other steps can be taken. If you have an airborne allergy, installing high-efficiency particulate air (HEPA) filters in your home and office is a good start, as they remove nearly 100 percent of pollens, molds, dust, and other irritants.

Medications, including antihistamines and decongestants, are a staple of allergy treatment, but they also have some unpleasant side effects (see chapter 9). Two commonly used antihistamines are dimenhydrinate (Benadryl) and diphenhydramine (Dramamine), which are helpful for people who experience dizziness related to allergies. Their most prominent side effect is drowsiness. The newest antihistamines are nonsedating and therefore do not cause drowsiness. Nasal steroidal inhalers are another effective way to block inhalant allergies with minimal side effects.

Immunotherapy in the form of allergy shots—injections of increasing concentrations of the offending allergens often taken regularly for years—can offer relief for some people.

Anemia

Anemia is a condition in which the number of red blood cells or the oxygen-carrying hemoglobin within them falls below optimal levels. This occurs either because your body is producing too few healthy red blood cells or because it's destroying them or losing them faster than it can replace them. Some of the most common symptoms associated with this blood disorder are dizziness, light-headedness, and fatigue. In fact, dizziness is frequently the first symptom people notice.

If you have anemia, you're not alone: approximately 3.5 million Americans of all ages suffer with some form of this disease. It's the most common blood disorder in the United States and affects mostly women and the elderly.

CAUSES OF ANEMIA

There are approximately 100 different types of anemia, so it's easy to understand why there can be many different causes. One of the most-recognized causes is an iron deficiency, which is why anemia is often referred to as "iron-poor blood." Anemia can also be caused by a vitamin deficiency (specifically, vitamin B12 and/or folic acid), loss of blood, chronic illness (e.g., cancer, AIDS, heart disease, rheumatoid arthritis, inflammatory bowel disease, and liver disease), or genetics (a hereditary disease or defect), or it can be a side effect of various medications.

HOW TO RECOGNIZE ANEMIA

In addition to the symptoms already mentioned, others associated with anemia include weakness, pale skin, rapid heartbeat, shortness of breath, numbness or coldness in the feet and hands, confusion, and chest pain. Left untreated, anemia can lead to serious complications, including irregular heart rhythm. In extreme cases, it can cause death.

Diagnosis and Treatment

Anemia is diagnosed with a physical examination, medical history, and blood tests, including a complete blood count (CBC), which measures the number of red blood cells and the amount of hemoglobin in your blood. Levels of specific nutrients, including iron, vitamin B12, and folic acid, also should be measured. Treatment will depend on the cause of the anemia. Nutritionally related anemia can be treated with supplements and dietary changes, but if an underlying disease is the cause, that disorder must be treated.

Chronic Fatigue and Immune Dysfunction Syndrome

When most people hear the terms chronic fatigue or chronic fatigue syndrome, they naturally—and rightfully—recognize that fatigue is the main symptom of this disorder. Fewer people probably realize that lightheadedness affects 75 percent of the people who have this conditio, and that dizziness affects 30 to 50 percent of them.

In 1984, more than 200 primarily young, wealthy, white women in one resort town fell victim to a mysterious illness that was characterized by severe fatigue, lightheadedness, muscle aches, and other symptoms. The media nicknamed the condition "Yuppie flu," and few people, including those in the medical profession, took the illness seriously. There were no tests to verify these symptoms, so most people thought the incident was just a fluke.

But it was not a fluke, and in 1988 the prestigious Centers for Disease Control and Prevention named the disease chronic fatigue syndrome. Today, it is uncertain exactly how many people have this illness, which is now called chronic fatigue and immune dysfunction syndrome (CFIDS), but estimates range from 800,000 to about 4 million in North America. By a three-to-one margin, more women than men are affected.

HOW TO RECOGNIZE CFIDS

Chronic fatigue and immune dysfunction syndrome can cause a wide range of symptoms that can affect any part of the body. In addition to overwhelming, consistent, debilitating fatigue and the other symptoms already mentioned, CFIDS is also characterized by swollen lymph nodes, painful joints, recurring headache, balance and coordination problems, difficulty looking at moving objects, short-term memory problems, blurred vision, depression, chills, shortness of breath, low-grade fever, sensitivity to heat and/or cold, numbness, tingling, fainting, ringing in the ears, and bowel problems.

Among teenagers with CFIDS, a form of chronic orthostatic intolerance called postural tachycardia syndrome (POTS; see chapter 6) is often seen. The main symptoms associated with POTS are dizziness, fatigue, nausea, abdominal pain, headache, shakiness, and difficulty thinking, symptoms that mimic those of CFIDS.

DIAGNOSIS AND TREATMENT

Because there are no specific tests to identify CFIDS and because its symptoms are so varied and are similar to those of many other disorders, CFIDS is difficult to diagnose. Basically, doctors must rule out other possible medical conditions before arriving at the diagnosis. Some health-care providers, however, do not even acknowledge that CFIDS exists, and some believe the symptoms are due to psychological or psychosomatic factors, including stress, anxiety, and depression.

JANET'S STORY

For about six months, Janet, a 27-year-old account executive, had been experiencing lightheadedness, dizziness, and feelings of "spaciness and disorientation" daily. These were accompanied by balance problems, particularly swaying when standing still. All of these symptoms were worse whenever she felt fatigued, which, Janet admitted, was happening more and more often lately. In fact, she confessed that there were days on which she had to drag herself out of bed to go to work and by noon she was exhausted. She had no energy to go out with her friends at night, and her work performance was suffering. By the time she came to my office, she was working part-time only, and even that was a struggle.

When we explored Janet's medical history, she told me the symptoms started a few weeks after she had gotten over a bad bout of the flu, about seven months ago. Before coming to me she had undergone an MRI scan prescribed by her primary care doctor, and it was normal. She had no personal or family history of any neurological or inner ear conditions, and she was not taking any medications.

Her physical and neurological examinations didn't reveal any problems, and she had no complaints of hearing loss, ringing in the ears, pressure in the ears, or vertigo. Her electronystagmography results were all normal. When we did the posturography test, she did demonstrate the excessive swaying she had mentioned to me. We ordered blood tests, which showed an Epstein-Barr viral infection, a possible indication of CFIDS.

For a short time we treated Janet with meclizine, a drug that helps suppress vertigo, but her symptoms worsened—as sometimes happens when people take this drug—so we discontinued it. Janet attended vestibular rehabilitation therapy sessions for two months and also continued with exercises at home as assigned to her by her therapist. Although her fatigue continued, she had great improvement in her balance and dizziness problems, and eventually she was able to return to work on a full-time basis.

Diabetes

Twelve percent of adults older than 40—that's the percentage of people who are believed to have the most common form of diabetes, noninsulin-dependent or type 2 diabetes, according to the American Diabetes Association. This disease is characterized either by an inability of the pancreas to produce a sufficient amount of insulin or by the body's inability to utilize the insulin it does manufacture. In people who have type 2 diabetes, dizziness and balance problems can be a frequent or even a common occurrence, depending on how well they manage their disease.

HOW TO RECOGNIZE DIABETES

Indications that you may have diabetes include an unexplained increase in appetite, unexplained weight loss, increased thirst, and frequent urination. Some people also experience dizziness, balance problems, nausea, fatigue, leg cramps, blurry vision, weakness, and persistent bladder or skin infections. Two important risk factors for diabetes are obesity (about 80 percent of people who have diabetes are overweight) and a family history of the disease.

Lightheadedness, dizziness, and balance problems in diabetes are often caused by low blood sugar (glucose) levels from overcorrecting the high glucose level, a condition known as hypoglycemia. (Balance and gait problems may also be associated with diabetic neuropathy, which is discussed in chapter 8 under "Neuropathy.") Other symptoms of hypoglycemia include confusion, irritability, and nervous habits. As diabetes progresses, blood flow is compromised; this can contribute to feelings of lightheadedness and episodes of orthostatic hypotension (see chapter 6).

HOW TO PREVENT HYPOGLYCEMIA

Hypoglycemia occurs in people who have diabetes for various reasons, including taking too much diabetes medication, consuming too little food compared with the amount of medication they've taken, skipping meals, emotional stress, drinking too much alcohol, excessive physical activity, or a combination of these factors. Thus preventing hypoglycemia begins by avoiding these triggers.

If you have diabetes, your health-care provider should teach you to recognize what triggers hypoglycemic attacks in you and the symptoms of the onset of such attacks. Regular monitoring of your blood sugar levels is one way to avoid such incidents. Talk to your doctor about how often you should check your blood sugar levels during the day. To prevent oncoming attacks, you should always have hard candy, dried fruit, or cookies with you. If you feel an attack coming on, you can eat these foods to get sugar into your body quickly.

Rheumatoid Arthritis

More than 2.5 million Americans have rheumatoid arthritis, an autoimmune disorder in which the immune system attacks the joints, and occasionally other parts of the body. This self-attack can have a significant impact on balance and coordination.

Rheumatoid arthritis is a progressive disease, so as time goes on, the bone and cartilage around the affected joints continue to deteriorate. There are several ways this deterioration can have a significant impact on balance. One way is when the disease affects the upper cervical spine (in the neck); this damages the joints and makes the neck area unstable, and this in turn causes balance and coordination problems.

Another way is when the rheumatoid arthritis affects the ankles, knees, and hips, making balance difficult. Some people also develop abnormal growths in their joints. These growths press against nerves and cause partial or complete loss of sensation or function in the affected body part, such as a foot. When signals from the joints are disrupted or go awry, balance is affected.

HOW TO RECOGNIZE RHEUMATOID ARTHRITIS

Rheumatoid arthritis is characterized by inflammation, pain, and stiffness in the joints, as well as limited mobility in the knuckles, wrists, hips, balls of the feet, knees, and other joints. It can also affect the spine.

But rheumatoid arthritis is more than a joint disease. This systemic disease also causes fever, fatigue, weight loss, and fragile skin that tends to bruise easily. Inflammation can also develop around the heart (inflammation of the pericardium), lymph nodes (lymphadenopathy), and spleen (splenomegaly). Anemia can also result from rheumatoid arthritis.

TREATMENT

Medical treatment of rheumatoid arthritis can include non-steroidal anti-inflammatory drugs (NSAIDs), which help reduce inflammation; disease-modifying antirheumatic drugs, which attempt to slow down the progression of the disease; and corti-costeroids and immunosuppressant drugs, which suppress the activity of the immune system and can slow bone destruction and control pain. All of these drugs have side effects, some of which are very serious (talk to your health-care practitioner about them), and some of these drugs cause dizziness (see chapter 9).

Vestibular rehabilitation therapy can be especially important for people who have rheumatoid arthritis, as this disease usually first becomes apparent in the prime years of their lives: 20 to 45. If rheumatoid arthritis has affected your balance or your ability to perform your job or everyday tasks, rehabilitation can be your ticket back to a more normal lifestyle. If you want to return to work or continue working, occupational therapists can provide balance and strength exercises and/or show you how to use devices that can assist you on the job and at home. Therapy is also helpful if you want to improve your ability to perform everyday activities such as walking, getting in and out of chairs and bed, and maintaining good balance to prevent falls.

Systemic Lupus Erythematosus

Systemic lupus erythematosus, also known as lupus or SLE, is a chronic disease in which nearly everyone affected—90 percent—has painful, inflamed arthritic joints that can send poor signals to the vestibular system. Thus an individual with lupus frequently has problems with balance and dizziness. Systemic lupus erythematosus is no small problem in this country: an estimated 1.5 million people in the United States have SLE, and 90 percent of them are women.

If you have lupus, you may also experience vertigo along with some hearing loss. Experts believe these symptoms are caused by inflammation of the blood vessels in the inner ear, which are commonly affected in this disease.

Lupus is truly systemic, because it can affect every part of the body—skin, organs, joints, and blood. Therefore its symptoms, in addition to those already mentioned, cover a wide spectrum:

rash, fatigue, heart problems, muscle weakness, anemia, fever, kidney inflammation, and seizures.

Unfortunately, there is no cure for lupus, so the main goal of treatment is to reduce inflammation, manage symptoms, and help prevent flare-ups. Typically this approach means patients take any number of drugs, including nonsteroidal anti-inflammatory drugs (NSAIDs) for muscle pain, inflammation, and arthritis; corticosteroids for inflammation; antimalarials (e.g., chloroquine [Aralen] or hydroxychloroquine [Plaquenil]) for skin and joint problems; and cytotoxic drugs (e.g., azathioprine [Imuran] and cyclophosphamide [Cytoxan]), to suppress the immune system and help reduce inflammation. Those who have problems with balance and coordination can benefit from vestibular rehabilitation therapy.

Thyroid Disorders

You may be surprised to learn that the thyroid—a gland located in the neck near the windpipe—produces a hormone that is critical for the normal development and function of the vestibular and auditory systems. This fact likely explains why some people who have hypothyroidism (low production of thyroid hormone) experience episodes of vertigo. It may also explain why some people who have Ménière's syndrome also have hypothyroidism.

THYROID AND THE INNER EAR

The inner ear is very sensitive to the level of thyroid hormone in the body, so fluctuations may cause dizziness and/or vertigo. This is especially important among women age 50 and older, because more than 10 percent of this population has symptoms of a thyroid problem—either too little hormone produced (hypothyroidism) or too much (hyperthyroidism). In addition to dizziness, hypothyroidism typically causes fatigue, inflammation, weight gain, dry flaky skin, sensitivity to cold, and depression, while hyperthyroidism can trigger weight loss.

Because thyroid problems are often overlooked in middle-aged women, it is up to you, if you are in this category and experiencing symptoms, to ask your health-care provider about undergoing thyroid tests.

DIAGNOSIS AND TREATMENT

Along with a physical examination and medical history, there are specific blood tests your doctor can order that can identify hypothyroidism. They include tests for:

- The amount of thyroxine (T4) secreted by the thyroid, as abnormally low levels suggest hypothyroidism.
- The level of thyroid-stimulating hormone (TSH) as high levels of this hormone are a very reliable test for hypothyroidism
- The level of the antithyroid peroxidase (TPO) antibody as high levels of this antibody are common in people who have hypothyroidism

Treatment of hypothyroidism consists of taking thyroid hormones, usually for the rest of your life. Because low or fluctuating thyroid hormone levels can cause dizziness and vertigo, it's important that you and your doctor find the best dose for you. Once a dose has been determined, you may subsequently need to return to your health-care practitioner for adjustments, because your medication needs can change due to stress, menopause, surgical procedures, serious or chronic illness, or physical trauma.

Polycythemia

Polycythemia is a blood disease in which there is an overproduction of red and white blood cells, as well as of platelets.

Symptoms typically come on slowly and include headache, dizziness, itchy skin (especially after taking a hot shower or bath), fullness in the left upper abdomen, fatigue, vision problems, shortness of breath, and red skin, especially on the face.

Treatment of polycythemia involves removal of about 1 pint of blood (phlebotomy) at regular intervals to reduce blood viscosity. This condition occurs in men more than in women, and 95 percent of the cases occur after age 40. Its cause is unknown.

Bottom Line

Dizziness, vertigo, and disequilibrium and the symptoms typically associated with them are frequently a part of the picture when it comes to systemic disorders. To get relief from these balance-related symptoms, it's necessary to be treated for the underlying medical condition. That being said, you should be aware that some of the medications your health-care practitioner may prescribe for you can cause side effects, including lightheadedness, dizziness, and disequilibrium, and you should ask if there are alternatives to those drugs. Also keep in mind that in some cases, vestibular rehabilitation therapy can be an integral part of your treatment program.

8

Visual and Sensory Disorders

The visual and proprioceptive systems play a significant role in balance, yet so far we haven't addressed disorders that specifically involve these two areas. In this chapter we explore the ailments and circumstances that change your ability to see and feel your environment fully, and how a disruption or distortion of vision and touch can have a big impact on balance. In the area of vision, we look at some disorders you may have heard about already, including cataracts, macular degeneration, and double vision. Other disorders have more unusual names, but their symptoms may seem more familiar once you read about them: ambient visual disorder, aneisokonia, and binocular vision dysfunction.

Next we'll look at sensory disorders, which for our purposes encompass three very significant areas: arthritis, which affects approximately 40 million Americans; peripheral neuropathy, a symptom that is associated with a number of disorders, especially diabetes; and aging, a natural fact of life which no one, who lives long enough, escapes.

Visual Disorders

Your visual system interacts intimately with your vestibular system, and both are involved in maintaining balance. In fact, about 20 percent of the nerve fibers in the eye interact directly with the vestibular system. So when something goes wrong with your vision, it's very possible you may also experience a problem with dizziness or balance.

For example, if you have ever had trouble getting used to a new pair of glasses, you've experienced the disharmony between what you see, and your sense of where you are and your attempt to maintain your balance. You may have felt dizzy for a few days or found yourself stepping up onto a curb, missing it completely, and losing your balance. Perhaps you had a headache for a day or so, felt dizzy when you looked down at the newspaper and then away from it, or experienced feelings of disorientation.

Problems adjusting to new glasses typically last only a few days as the brain gradually compensates and adjusts for the new signals coming in. If you don't notice significant improvement after a few days, however, you should return to your optician or opthalmologist to see if there is something wrong with your prescription.

In addition to getting new glasses, there are some visual disorders that can cause dizziness and balance problems. You should consult your opthalmologist as soon as possible if you think you have any of these conditions or if you are experiencing other visual problems (see the box on page 132).

AMBIENT VISUAL DISORDER

Vision is the result of many processes, and one of them is called ambient process, which provides information to your brain about where you are in space and thus helps you maintain balance and coordination. This process often malfunctions after a stroke or an injury to the brain, which can cause individuals to experience dizziness and balance problems such as a tendency to lean to either side, backward, or forward. This vision problem can often be treated by wearing glasses that contain special prisms or partial patches, along with vestibular rehabilitation therapy as needed.

ANEISOKONIA

The magnification of images often differs between the eyes, but for some people the difference is excessive. This condition is known as aneisokonia, and it can cause eyestrain, dizziness, headache, and disorientation. Aneisokonia can be corrected using special eyeglass lenses called isokonic lenses.

BINOCULAR VISION DYSFUNCTION

The ability to see with both eyes requires that the eyes and brain work together in synch. Occasionally, however, injury, illness, or some unknown factor will cause the eyes to weaken and overreact. When this happens, the eyes tend to drift outward (toward the ears) or inward (toward the nose). This results in double vision, muscle spasms, eyestrain, and excessive peripheral (side) visual stimulation, which triggers balance problems and dizziness. Treatment includes the use of special eyeglass lenses, prisms included in eyeglasses, and eye exercises.

CATARACTS

A cataract is a clouding of the crystalline lens, which lies behind the pupil of the eye. The purpose of the lens is to help focus light on the retina, which is at the back of the eye. If the lens becomes cloudy, light that enters the eye cannot reach the retina properly, and so vision becomes blurry. Some people also experience a loss of contrast and double vision, which can lead to balance problems.

Cataracts frequently accompany aging; in fact, more than 50

percent of people older than 65 have some cataract development. Cataracts also may occur because of an eye injury or chronic eye disease or as a symptom of another disease, such as diabetes.

Cataracts may develop over a few months or several years; they may grow until they reach a certain point and stop progressing, or continue to get worse. Because there are no medications known that can stop the disease process, surgery is the only effective way to treat it. During surgery, the cataract is removed and an artificial lens (intraocular lens) is implanted.

More than 1 million cataract procedures are performed in the United States every year, most without significant complications. Postoperative infection is possible and is characterized by dizziness, headache, muscle aches, and fever. If these symptoms occur, see your physician immediately.

DOUBLE VISION

Double vision (also known as diplopia) can be a seriously debilitating condition, as it can prevent people from driving, working, or getting around safely, especially in the elderly. The condition occurs when both eyes fail to work together, resulting in one eye turning in, out, up, or down when compared with the other eye. Double vision often causes dizziness and balance problems. Treatment can include the use of special eyeglass lenses that act as a patch, prisms included in glasses, and surgery.

GLAUCOMA

More than 3 million Americans have glaucoma, an eye disease which can eventually lead to blindness. Glaucoma is actually a term for a group of diseases that involve elevated pressure inside the eye. The pressure typically causes no pain, but it damages the optic nerve, a bundle of nerve fibers that is necessary for good vision.

As the disease progresses, people may notice they have lost

peripheral vision or they have difficulty focusing on close objects. They may see halos around lights and need to change their eyeglass prescription frequently. These symptoms are frequently accompanied by feelings of lightheadedness or unsteadiness as their vision becomes more unreliable. The risk of losing their balance and falling increases as their vision decreases. Eventually, their sight may be gone completely.

The best way to beat this eye disease is to have regular eye exams and to be checked for glaucoma. If glaucoma is caught early, the inner eye pressure can be controlled and the risk of blindness can be eliminated. Typically, health-care providers prescribe eyedrops or oral medication designed either to cause the eyes to produce less fluid or to help drain excess fluid from the eye. Another treatment option is laser surgery (laser trabeculoplasty), which helps drain fluid from the eye. Surgery is usually performed after medications have been tried; in many cases medications are still needed after surgery.

MACULAR DEGENERATION

Among people 65 years and older, macular degeneration is the primary cause of new blindness. This common eye disease gradually (in most cases) destroys sharp, central vision, which is processed by the central part of the retina, or macula. The initial symptoms include slightly blurry vision that slowly becomes worse over time. If only one eye is affected, you may not notice the blurriness because the healthy eye will compensate. Eventually, however, the blurry vision will become noticeable, and dizziness, disorientation, and problems with balance may develop as vision grows worse. As the macula becomes damaged, tasks that require looking straight ahead, such as reading, driving, and watching television, become increasingly difficult.

Two forms of macular degeneration exist: dry and wet. The dry form affects about 90 percent of the estimated 3.6 million

Americans who have the disease. In the wet form, the first symptoms include seeing wavy lines where there are straight ones (e.g., the vertical lines on a paneled wall or the dividing lines in the road may look crooked) and decreasing central vision. This visual distortion can cause dizziness, unsteadiness, and loss of balance. Unlike the dry form, wet macular degeneration usually progresses rapidly and can eventually cause blindness.

Currently there is no treatment for the dry form of macular degeneration, but there are several treatments that have proved helpful for the wet variety. Laser surgery (laser photocoagulation) can be used to seal the abnormal leaking blood vessels in the retina; photodynamic therapy injects a dye which, when exposed to the laser, seals leaky vessels. Neither of these approaches can repair damage that has already occurred, and in many cases they simply slow the progression of the disease.

DO YOU HAVE A VISION PROBLEM?

You should see your ophthalmologist if you experience any of the following symptoms. Also don't fail to mention them to your health-care practitioner when you provide him or her with your medical history.

- Dizziness, headache, and/or nausea after reading
- Having to tilt your head in order to see reading material or objects
- Itchy, sore, and/or red eyes
- Jerky eye movements
- One eye's turning in or out
- Excessive blinking, squinting, or eye rubbing
- Needing to close or block one eye when reading

Neuropathy

Neuropathy (also known as peripheral [away from the spinal cord and brain] neuropathy or sensory peripheral neuropathy) is a painful condition in which there has been damage to the peripheral nerves. In healthy individuals, the peripheral nerves send messages to the spinal cord, which then sends them along to the brain, which informs people where their hands, legs, arms, and feet are in relation to the rest of their environment. But for many people, damaged nerves inhibit those messages, causing these people to lose their ability to sense where they are in their environment, and they can lose their balance.

HOW TO RECOGNIZE NEUROPATHY

Neuropathy can be caused by more than 100 different factors including alcoholism (see chapter 9), diabetes (see pp. 134–136), exposure to chemicals or heavy metals, infections, poor circulation to the feet, nutritional deficiencies, or pressure from a fracture or another type of trauma that causes signals not to be transmitted or to be translated properly.

Regardless of the cause, people who have injured or damaged peripheral nerves experience similar symptoms. Often the first symptom is tingling in the fingers, toes, or both. Over time, the tingling spreads through the hands or feet and can transform into a burning or prickling sensation. These feelings may be constant or intermittent, mild to severe, and even debilitating to the point where the people can't touch or place any pressure on their feet or hands. Even a breeze blowing on their hand or foot may be unbearable.

In contrast, some people lose all sensation in their feet, hands, legs, or arms. When this happens, they may injure themselves and not realize it. When they can't properly feel the ground beneath their feet, it is difficult for them to walk or to maintain their balance.

NEUROPATHY AND THE ELDERLY

In the Women's Health and Aging Study, 58 percent of women showed evidence of neuropathy by age 65. Peripheral neuropathy is of special concern among older adults, because it is associated with unsteadiness and a high percentage of falls. About one-third of elderly Americans fall each year, and 5 percent or more of these falls result in a fracture, at a cost of more than $12 billion per year. These numbers do not include those who suffer pain and discomfort, without fractures, from these falls, the cost these falls have on the individuals due to their inability to do everyday tasks and maintain independence.

DIABETIC NEUROPATHY

One of the most significant causes of neuropathy is diabetes. Although people who have diabetes can develop neuropathy at any time, signs of nerve problems typically appear within the first ten years of their receiving a diagnosis of diabetes. Individuals who have type 1 diabetes run the most risk of serious neuropathy, as they have diabetes longer than those who get the type 2 form. Overall, about 60 percent of the people who have diabetes have neuropathy.

The exact cause of diabetic neuropathy is not known, but factors that appear to play a part include:

- Heredity. Some genetic traits may predispose some people to be more susceptible to nerve problems.
- High blood sugar levels. An elevated level of sugar (glucose) in the bloodstream causes chemical changes in nerves and hinders their ability to transmit signals. Glucose can also damage blood vessels and prevent them from providing proper nutrition to the nerves.

In addition to the symptoms mentioned above (loss of sensation, tingling, prickling, burning, all of which can cause balance problems), diabetic neuropathy can also affect the nerves that serve the internal organs or even specific nerves and cause dizziness, fainting, indigestion, diarrhea, constipation, bladder infections, double vision, hearing problems, severe lower back pain, impotence, excessive sweating, and pain in the chest, stomach, or flank.

HAROLD'S STORY

"I'm unsteady on my feet, doc, and I'm too young for this to be happening." These were the first words Harold, a 47-year-old convenience store owner, said to me the first time we met at my office.

Harold told me that he had had insulin-dependent diabetes for nearly 30 years and that he was afraid his balance problems might be related to his disease. For the past six months, he had been experiencing numbness and tingling in both feet almost daily, and it got worse when his feet were cold. He also noted that sometimes at night, his feet would burn and make it difficult for him to sleep. The only other symptom he mentioned was that he found it difficult to maneuver in poorly lit places.

During testing, I noticed that Harold had reduced sensation in both legs below the knees. When he tried standing on a soft, foam surface, he couldn't do so with his eyes open or closed. During computerized platform posturography, he demonstrated excessive swaying. When I did the reflex test of his ankles, there were no ankle jerks, which indicated that Harold had poor nerve function in his ankles. Examination of his eyes suggested diabetic retinopathy, a common and serious condition among people who have diabetes in which vision can deteriorate and eventually result in blindness. His electronystagmography results were normal, suggesting that he had no problems with his vestibular system.

I explained to Harold that his balance symptoms were likely related to diabetic neuropathy and diabetic retinopathy; this meant that he had reduced function in two (proprioceptive and visual) out of three systems needed for balance. I recommended that he begin vestibular rehabilitation therapy where therapists could help him with gait and balance training exercises and teach him how to use a cane, which would give him more sensory input to make up for the reduced sensations from his feet and ankles.

Harold completed several months of vestibular rehabilitation therapy and improved enough so that he is more confident when walking on various types of surfaces and feels more secure about his ability to keep working for many more years.

OTHER TYPES OF NEUROPATHY

In addition to diabetic neuropathy, some of the other more common types include the following:

Alcoholic Neuropathy. Between 25 and 30 percent of the people who suffer with neuropathy abuse alcohol. Alcoholic neuropathy is caused by a vitamin deficiency (B vitamins in particular) related to excessive intake of alcohol (see "Alcohol, Caffeine, and Nicotine" in chapter 9). Symptoms of alcoholic neuropathy usually begin in the feet and then move to the legs. Occasionally the arms are affected as well. Numbness and painful tingling can make it difficult or impossible to walk or maintain balance. Besides a vitamin deficiency, alcohol alone may have a toxic effect on the nervous system.

Kidney Disease. People who have chronic kidney (renal) failure often have neuropathy. The symptoms typically include cramping and numbness that start in the feet and progress slowly up the legs. Once patients begin renal dialysis, which helps the body rid itself of toxins, symptoms usually subside.

Cancer. Cancer can cause neuropathy in several ways. One way is through tumors that spread and affect the nerves; another is through the release of substances from certain types of cancers that can cause nerve damage. This latter type of neuropathy is characterized by aching pain in the legs and arms, problems with balance and walking, and weakness.

TREATMENT FOR NEUROPATHY

Your health-care provider will treat your neuropathy on the basis of several factors, including your age, medical history, the severity of your disease, and how well you can tolerate specific medications or therapies. The goal is not only to get you relief from pain but to prevent further nerve damage and to maintain functioning.

Treatment may include pain medication, stress reduction techniques (e.g., hypnosis, biofeedback, meditation, and relaxation training), or transcutaneous electronic nerve stimulation (TENS), a form of therapy in which harmless electric impulses are transmitted through the skin via electrodes. Electric stimulation of the nerves blocks the pain signals before they reach the brain. The stimulation is delivered by a credit-card-sized device that patients can wear on their belt at all times for continuous relief. Vestibular rehabilitation therapy can be pursued along with other therapies to help build strength and balance.

Aging

Although there are some inspiring exceptions, most of us lose function throughout the body as we age. Depending on factors such as heredity, lifestyle, and environmental influences, some of us experience more functional loss and susceptibility to disease than others. Part of the decline in function involves the three systems that make up balance—visual, vestibular, and proprioceptive—as well as the brain.

In many older people, the decline in function is subtle, gradual, and taken in stride. But for others, their way of life undergoes dramatic changes. Forty percent of people 60 years and older experience episodes of dizziness that seriously affect their daily activities. If you are among this population, you know how distressing dizziness is in your life. But why does it happen?

COMMON DECLINES OF AGING

Researchers have established that in order for us to maintain equilibrium, it's necessary for at least two of the three main sensory systems to work properly and provide accurate information to the brain. As we age, there is a significant increase in the chance that some portion of any of these systems will function less than optimally. Sometimes the decline in function is the result of damage or injury, but in many cases it's simply the result of degenerative changes that commonly occur as we age.

Although the decline in function of individual areas or organs may be minor for many older adults, it can be enough to cause lightheadedness, dizziness, or balance problems. In some cases, it is the accumulation of declines in various parts of the body that results in a loss of balance. These problems with disequilibrium are not rare: approximately 12.5 million Americans older than 65 have a dizziness or balance disorder that interferes significantly with their lives.

Here are some of the common functional losses that occur with aging.

- Blood flow to the inner ear declines.
- Nerve fibers, hair cells, the utricle, and the saccule degenerate, and do not repair.
- The ability of the vestibular nerve to transmit signals declines.
- The number of nerve cells in the brain stem declines; this appears to be responsible for the difficulties elderly people have in compensating for some inner ear disorders.

- There's a gradual loss of cells in the motor and sensory areas of the brain.
- Healthy elderly men tend to take shorter steps and swing their arms less than when they were younger. The gait of healthy elderly women, tends to have a waddling effect.
- Visual acuity (the ability to discriminate the fine details of objects) declines in some people and can contribute to instability, fear, and anxiety when walking, which can increase the risk of falling
- Muscle strength in the legs and trunk decreases; this may result in a decline in the ability to maintain equilibrium
- Feedback from the joints and muscles of the legs decreases; this results in decreased coordination and balance.
- Posture changes; specifically the center of gravity tends to shift forward. This results in more body weight on the toes and thus a greater risk of falling forward.

In addition, older adults are more likely to be taking several medications. Between ages 55 and 65, for example, individuals are typically given an average of eight different prescriptions during any given year. Among people older than 70, an average of six and a half drugs are taken daily. The Food and Drug Administration reports that the average older person takes two over-the-counter drugs daily in addition to prescription medications. Very often, the drugs older people are taking are for conditions such as high blood pressure, depression, heart conditions, and diabetes. It just so happens that drugs in these categories are often associated with side effects such as dizziness and balance problems. Thus frequently older people who go to a doctor complaining of dizziness or balance problems find that their problem, or at least part of it, can be attributed to the medications they are taking for other problems. In chapter 9, we take a closer look at the role of medications in dizziness and balance problems and explain which drugs can cause these symptoms.

FALLS AND DISEQUILIBRIUM

According to the American Academy of Orthopedic Surgeons, 30 percent of the people older than age 65 will fall each year. The risk of falls increases with age, and it is greater in women than in men. Falls are the leading cause of injury among older adults and are the number one cause of accidental death in people older than 85. Overall, about 20 percent of Americans between the ages of 65 and 75 have a balance disorder, and by age 75, that figure is 25 percent. Treatment of fall-related injuries, including fractures, costs more than $20 billion per year, according to the American Academy of Orthopedic Surgeons. (See "Steps to Prevent Age-Related Dizziness and Falls" in chapter 12.)

Why do older adults fall? As we've already mentioned, natural age-related declines in the functioning of the vestibular, visual, and proprioceptive systems are significant factors. To this can be added any damage or injuries related to illness or disease, such as diabetes, Parkinson's disease, glaucoma, macular degeneration, peripheral neuropathy, or any number of inner ear disorders.

ROBERT'S STORY

"I've lost my balance. I can't walk straight any more." These were the first words out of Robert's mouth when he initially came to see me. At 83 years young, Robert prided himself on being self-reliant, and his gradual decline in walking ability had him very upset. While sitting and lying down he felt fine, but when he got up to walk, he said, "I walk like a drunk."

A visit to his primary care physician hadn't shown anything unusual. Robert had a slight hearing loss in both ears and high blood pressure that he kept under control with medication and he was taking cardiac drugs, but he was okay in all other respects. He told me he had never experienced any vertigo, ringing in his ears, or fullness in his ears.

When I conducted my examination I found some degenerative changes in hearing associated with his age, reduced responses on balance testing, and difficulty maintaining balance on the posturography test. All of these findings are common among elderly people. I explained to Robert that there was normal, age-related deterioration in his balance system that made his inner ear less sensitive when responding to balance stimuli. This meant that both his acceptance of stimulation and his response to it were slower. So when he walked on an uneven surface, the receptors in his feet and ankles were not as quick to pick up the different pressures, and his brain responded slower to the signals it did receive.

Robert immediately wanted to know if there was a pill he could take to help correct this problem, and I assured him that medication would only make the problem worse, plus it would make him more tired and could cause mental confusion. I recommended he attend vestibular rehabilitation therapy to work on ways to compensate for his unsteadiness and to learn some important tips on how to avoid falling. He followed my advice and did notice some improvement in his ability to walk. In particular, strength exercises for his legs were helpful, and attending the sessions also improved his confidence and mood. I also suggested he learn tai chi, a system of Chinese movement exercises that can improve balance (see chapter 12, "Vestibular Rehabilitation and Other Physical Therapies").

Osteoarthritis

Wear and tear, these are the words often associated with osteoarthritis, a painful condition that affects approximately 40 million Americans. That wear and tear also has the effect of causing a loss of sensation in the joints of many people, and that loss can result in problems with balance.

When we talk about wear and tear, we're describing how the cartilage (the tough, shock-absorbing tissue that secretes a thick fluid which prevents bones from grinding together) wears away, so that the bones rub together. This motion allows painful bone spurs to develop. In some joints, excess fluid may accumulate, which causes swelling. In others, there may be too little fluid, which causes stiffness.

OSTEOARTHRITIS AND BALANCE

When you consider all the damage that occurs in osteoarthritis, it's easy to understand why people with this disease experience pain, limited movement and flexibility, and inflammation. Because their joints are affected, they also experience a proprioceptive loss (loss of a sense of where the joint is in space) and thus may lose their balance and coordination. Especially among people who have osteoarthritis of the knee (a very common condition among older adults), there is knee pain, a loss of strength in the quadriceps muscle (muscle in the thigh which helps stabilize the knee), and a decrease in joint mobility, which can result in unsteadiness and falls. A comprehensive physical therapy program is necessary to help improve muscle strength and thus stabilize the knee.

CAUSES AND TREATMENT

An estimated 80 percent of people who have osteoarthritis are 65 years old or older, yet osteoarthritis is not an inevitable part of the aging process. Risk factors for the disease include heredity, history of a severe or recurrent joint injury, being overweight, living in a cold climate, and excessive exercise (prolonged participation in activities that place a great deal of stress on the joints, such as long-distance running or football).

Fortunately, most people who have osteoarthritis experience only mild or moderate symptoms and treat themselves with over-the-counter medications and natural supplements. An estimated 16 million Americans, however, experience progressively worsening symptoms and eventually become disabled.

Treatment typically consists of anti-inflammatory drugs (e.g., ibuprofen, indomethacin, and others, all of which may worsen joint destruction by preventing the formation of healthy tissue in the joints), acetaminophen (a noninflammatory pain reliever such as Tylenol), glucosamine sulfate (a natural remedy that reduces inflammation and may help build cartilage), and chondroitan (another natural remedy that helps bring fluid into cartilage and thus reduce wear and tear). All of these treatments are available over-the-counter.

Bottom Line

When the sensory receptors in the visual and proprioceptive systems cannot and do not send complete or appropriate signals to the central nervous system, the result can be a loss of balance, incoordination, lightheadedness, or dizziness. The disruption of these signals is especially troublesome for elderly people, who are prone to falls and fractures. In order to correct the problems with balance and dizziness, it's necessary to treat the underlying conditions. In many cases, doctors suggest their patients participate in vestibular rehabilitation therapy as well, as it can improve balance, self-confidence, and quality of life.

9

Drugs and Environmental Causes

We live in an increasingly toxic world. It seems that everywhere we turn—at work, at home, in school, and at play—there are substances that can cause us harm. Whether we consume, absorb, or otherwise expose ourselves to these substances willingly or unwillingly, they have the power to cause lightheadedness, dizziness, vertigo, unsteadiness, incoordination, and other associated symptoms. A better awareness of these substances, the effects they can have on you, and how to avoid them is important if you want to avoid dizziness and balance problems.

These toxic substances fall into two categories. In one category are those we typically ingest intentionally, including some common over-the-counter and prescription medications, alcohol, caffeine, and nicotine. In the other category are insidious environmental influences, especially pollution and toxins found in the air, water, soil, food, and common objects we use or come into contact with in our daily lives.

The substances in both these categories have two things in common, namely, their ability to negatively affect your nervous system and cause the symptoms we've just mentioned and the fact that they are often overlooked as causing or contributing to dizziness and disequilibrium. That's why in the next few pages we want you to learn more about these toxins so you can better work with your health-care providers to uncover whether any of them may be a cause of your balance problems.

Drugs That Can Make You Dizzy

It's sad but true: the very medications we often take to help us feel better can also cause other symptoms, sometimes ones that are worse than the symptoms we were treating originally. It's also true that many times, health-care providers fail to tell their patients about the side effects they can expect from their medications.

Another truism is that many common medications can cause lightheadedness, dizziness, vertigo, and imbalance. In fact, drug-induced dizziness is one of the main causes of dizziness in the United States. And one final fact: some of the very same drugs your doctor may prescribe to *treat* dizziness can in fact *cause* dizziness if taken beyond a few days or weeks, depending on the medication.

IS IT A DRUG OR A DISEASE?

Symptoms of dizziness, imbalance, vertigo, hearing loss, and ringing in the ears associated with drug use are similar to those caused by the diseases discussed elsewhere in this book. When we talk about drugs and chemicals that can cause these symptoms, we're talking about *ototoxicity* (oto means "ear," and toxicity means "poisoning"). (Chemicals and environmental toxins are discussed separately below.)

Some drugs are poisonous to the hair cells in the inner ear (in both the cochlea and the vestibular areas) or to the vestibulo-cochlear nerve (the nerve that sends balance and hearing signals from the inner ear to the brain). That's why in many cases, people who take these drugs experience both balance and hearing problems. In fact, the word *ototoxicity* refers to both vestibular and hearing problems caused by medications and chemicals.

Depending on the drug used, heredity, other medication use, and many other factors, a drug may cause temporary or permanent effects. Fortunately, most people who experience ototoxicity have only temporary symptoms or minor permanent damage. Even so, any damage can be disruptive to your life, and there is always the risk of more serious permanent damage. Therefore, you should always consult your physician immediately if you are experiencing any symptoms associated with drug use.

The symptoms of ototoxicity can be mild to severe, they can occur rapidly or slowly, and they can be found in one or both ears. If you have a slow loss of inner function in one ear only, you will likely experience mild symptoms that disappear in a day or two, while a sudden, rapid loss in one ear may produce vertigo, vomiting, and nystagmus that are debilitating enough to keep you in bed for several days.

If, however, you have serious damage to both ears, symptoms may include headache, disequilibrium so severe you can't walk or tolerate moving your head, severe fatigue, and blurry vision. After you discontinue taking the drug and undergo vestibular rehabilitation therapy, you can expect some recovery of your balance function, although you will likely continue to experience some problems with equilibrium.

DIAGNOSING OTOTOXICITY

Because there are no specific tests for ototoxicity, an accurate diagnosis depends on the patient's history, symptoms, and test results, but especially on the history. Individuals must tell their health-care providers about any and all medications they have taken recently or are currently taking. Tests, including electronystagmography, computerized platform posturography, the rotary chair test, the auditory brain stem response test, and audiograms, can only reveal the extent of damage that has been done, not the drug that caused it.

HOW COMMON IS OTOTOXICITY?

This is a good question, but no clear answer can be given. The Food and Drug Administration (FDA) doesn't require drug manufacturers to determine the effects a new drug may have on inner ear function or structure when they are testing new drugs for safety. Typically, the FDA, medical experts, or the general public discover that a drug causes ototoxicity only after enough people take the drug and experience the symptoms, and then complain to their health-care providers, the FDA, and other authorities. This is how drugs like aspirin, streptomycin, and quinine were discovered to be ototoxic—after they were approved for general use and people became ill from using them.

GETTING DRUG SMART

Your best defense against drug-induced dizziness or balance problems is to be a cautious consumer. Educate yourself about any medications you are taking, both over-the-counter and prescription. Ask your health-care provider or pharmacist for complete information about the side effects of your medications. You can also refer to one of many consumer drug guides, available in libraries and bookstores (see Suggested Readings).

To get you started, we've provided a list of some of the more common drugs that can cause lightheadedness, dizziness, vertigo, and/or imbalance (see the box). The list presents categories of drugs (e.g., antianxiety drugs and diuretics), with examples of specific medications within each category. This list is not exhaustive; there may be other drugs within each category that also cause these symptoms. Ask your health-care provider about the drugs you are taking.

DRUGS THAT CAN CAUSE SYMPTOMS OF BALANCE DISORDERS

ANTIANXIETY DRUGS

- Buspirone (BuSpar) and butalbital combinations (Fioricet with codeine).

ANTIBIOTICS (NONAMINOGLYCOSIDES)

- Vancomycin (Vancocin and Vancoled). Should be a treatment of last resort as it can permanently damage the inner ear, although its effects are more reversible than those of gentamicin (see antibiotics). Also in this category are erythromycin and polymyxin B.

ANTIBIOTICS (AMINOGLYCOSIDES)

- Amikacin, dihydrostreptomycin, gentamicin, kanamycin, neomycin, netilmicin, ribostamycin, and tobramycin. Should be used as a treatment of last resort, as they can cause permanent damage to the inner ear.

ANTICANCER DRUGS

- Cisplatin (Platinol). Can damage hair cells in the inner ear and also cause permanent hearing loss. Cyclophosphamide (Cytoxan) is also in this category.

ANTICONVULSANTS

- Carbamazepine (Tegretol).

ANTIDEPRESSANTS

- Amitriptyline (Elavil) and paroxetine (Paxil).

ASPIRIN

- Aspirin, and other salicylates. Likely to cause ringing in the ears and hearing loss (both reversible) at high doses (greater than 2,700 milligrams per day).

DIABETES DRUGS

- Glimepiride (Amaryl) and glipizide (Glucotrol).

ANTIHISTAMINES

- Clemastine fumarate (Tavist), cyproheptadine (Periactin), diphenhydramine (Benadryl), and promethazine (Phenergan).

ANTIMALARIAL DRUGS

- Quinine, chloroquine, and quinidine; also quinine (tonic) water. More likely to cause ringing in the ears and hearing loss (both reversible) than dizziness; however, dizziness can occur.

ANTIRHEUMATIC DRUGS

- Methotrexate (Methotrexate [MTX] and Rheumatex).

ANTIULCER DRUGS

- Cimetidine (Tagamet).

DIURETICS (WATER PILLS)

- Furosemide (Lasix), bumetamide (Bumex), and torsemide (Demadex). Associated more with ringing in the ears and hearing loss (both reversible once the drug is stopped) than with dizziness, but the latter does occur on occasion.

HEART DISEASE DRUGS

- Carvedilol (Coreg), carteolol (Cartrol), and nicardipine (Cardene).

HIGH BLOOD PRESSURE DRUGS

- Captopril (Capoten), methyldopa (Aldomet), propranolol (Inderal), ramipril (Altace), and reserpine (Serpasil).

MUSCLE RELAXANTS

- Carisoprodol (Soma).

NARCOTICS

- Oxycodone/acetaminophen (Percocet) and oxycodone (OxyContin).

NICOTINE (AS A SMOKING DETERRENT)

- Nicoderm (transdermal patch).

NONSTEROIDAL ANTI-INFLAMMATORY DRUGS (NSAIDs)

- Ibuprofen (Advil and Motrin), indomethacin (Indocin), and naproxen (Aleve). Can cause ringing in the ears and hearing loss (both reversible) at high doses (greater than 2,700 milligrams per day). The biggest concern with this category of drugs is that most of them are available over-the-counter, so many people tend to regard them as less potent than prescription drugs. Thus more people have a tendency to take higher doses of them.

TREATMENT

The type of symptom you experience with ototoxicity dictates the type of treatment that's best to relieve it. Vestibular rehabilitation therapy is effective for those who have experienced a loss of balance (see chapter 12). Certain exercises can be done to help the brain compensate for the changed information it receives from the damaged inner ear. People who experience hearing loss can benefit from hearing aids or, in severe cases, cochlear implants.

Environmental Causes

What price do we pay for progress? That's a question more and more people are asking, as it becomes increasingly obvious that many of the substances—especially chemicals and heavy metals found in products we use everyday—developed and produced in the name of progress are responsible for or contribute to many of our medical problems. Dizziness and difficulties with balance are among them.

Chemicals spew into our atmosphere from factory smoke stacks and vehicles on road and rail; discharge spills into our waterways from factories; fertilizers, pesticides, and animal waste run off from farms are in our soil and water; chemically treated furniture, building materials, toys, clothing, and hundreds of other everyday items are in our homes—the list could go on and on.

Most of our fruits, vegetables, and grains are sprayed with poisons; animals raised for meat are injected with antibiotics, steroids, and hormones; and our water supply is treated with chemicals. Many people spray their lawns and trees with chemicals and have exterminators come into their homes to spread another layer of toxins (see box). The assault is from every direction, and many of the attackers can have an effect on our health in general and our balance in particular. Why? Because these poisons are neurotoxins—substances that are poisonous to the nervous system.

DANGEROUS COMMON PESTICIDES STILL ON THE MARKET

If you're a home gardener, landscaper, or golfer or if you work for a lawn and garden store, landscaper, groundskeeper, or golf course or if you treat your house for common pests, take note. In December 2000, the Environmental Protection Agency announced that over the next four years, the common home and garden insecticide called diazinon would be phased out because it causes various neurological effects. Short-term effects include dizziness, headache, nausea, swollen joints, disorientation, and respiratory problems, while long-term exposure can seriously damage body functions.

Diazinon is used to control pests in the soil, on ornamental plants, and in fruit orchards and vegetable fields. It is also used to control household pests such as flies, cockroaches, and fleas.

Diazinon is one of more than 40 members of the pesticide family known as organophosates. Diazinon's "cousins" are still on the market, many of them in commonly used home pest management products, and all with the ability to cause the same symptoms as diazinon. Young children are especially susceptible to these symptoms because their organ systems are still developing. Products that contain diazinon include Dexol Diazinon Spray, Hot Shots, No Pest, Real-Kill, Ortho Diazinon Granules, and Spectracide.

MULTIPLE CHEMICAL SENSITIVITY

Although it is not universally accepted among those in the medical community as a physical disorder, multiple chemical sensitivity is very real to millions of people. Multiple chemical sensitivity is a condition in which the body reacts strongly and negatively to a wide range of substances, as diverse as perfume and cigarette smoke, plastics and newspaper print. According to the American Chemical Society, multiple chemical sensitivity strongly affects 2 to 5 percent of the people and moderately impacts 10 to 15 percent.

People with multiple chemical sensitivity cannot tolerate even minimal exposure to certain chemicals that normally don't bother most people or that trouble them only mildly. It is believed this intolerance is the result of a genetic malfunction that prevents the production of enzymes that normally metabolize the toxins and neutralize the damage they can do.

The litany of symptoms related to multiple chemical sensi-tivities makes it clear that this health condition is a threat to bal-ance and well-being: fatigue, vision problems, hearing problems, dizziness, nausea, sleep disorders, depression, memory difficul-ties, problems thinking, chest pain, muscle aches, joint pain, and rashes, among others. Not everyone with multiple chemical sen-sitivity experiences all of these symptoms.

A diagnosis of multiple chemical sensitivity can be difficult to reach, but if you suspect you have this condition, you can greatly help your health-care practitioner if you keep a diary of your diet, exposure to different chemicals and situations, and how you react to them. A knowledgeable doctor can then make a diagnosis using this information along with a thorough physical examination; a detailed medical history; analyses of blood, urine, hair, and fatty tissue for chemical levels; and a liver function test to determine whether the organ is properly clearing toxins from your body. (For more information about multiple chemical sensi-tivities, see appendix C, Resources.)

SICK-BUILDING SYNDROME

Sick-building syndrome is a situation in which individuals who work or live in a specific building experience acute health prob-lems that are associated with being in that building. These symp-toms disappear—sometimes gradually, sometimes abruptly—once the people leave the building.

Patricia is a 47-year-old software designer who noticed symp-toms her first day on her new job. At first she chalked up the dizziness, nausea, difficulty concentrating, and throat irritation to an unfortunate bout of the flu combined with "new job jitters." After two weeks, however, she felt no better and, in fact, learned that most of her coworkers were experiencing similar ill effects, plus eye irritation, dry cough, itchy skin, and fatigue. Patricia then found out that just a week before she started her new posi-tion, the office manager had hired a new cleaning company that came in once a week to do the floors and carpets. The chemicals used by the company lingered in the office, and Patricia and her office mates were suffering the ill effects.

The office manager decided to change cleaning services and switched to an environmentally responsible one. Within a month, everyone's symptoms had subsided a great deal, although it was several months before Patricia felt 100 percent better.

Patricia was fortunate, because many sick-building-syndrome situations do not end as well. In many cases, the cause of the problem is not found. In most cases, indoor air pollution is the problem. Many people don't realize that common items such as adhesives, carpeting, copy machines, drapes, manufactured wood products (e.g., furniture), upholstery, and plastics emit toxic chemicals into the air. Those, along with more obvious toxins—pesticides used to control indoor pests, paints, solvents, and cleaning agents—can cause sick-building syndrome because they emit volatile organic compounds, such as formaldehyde.

Other sources of contaminants that can cause sick-building syndrome include pollen, viruses, molds, and bacteria, which can breed in standing water that can collect in humidifiers and ducts or that may have collected in ceiling tiles, carpet, or insulation. One factor that contributed to sick-building syndrome was the trend started in the late 1970s toward building buildings that were more airtight in an effort to conserve energy. This step led to poorer ventilation in many buildings. Efforts have been made in recent years to improve ventilation in new buildings to help prevent this health problem.

HEAVY METALS AND OTOTOXICITY

Among the dozens of toxins we are exposed to, two of the most common ones are mercury and lead. Both of these heavy metals can be inhaled or ingested easily, and once in the body, they have no problem moving into the brain and attacking the central nervous system. That's when the problems begin.

Mercury toxicity, for example, causes fatigue, blurry vision, balance problems, dizziness, hearing loss, insomnia, tingling sensations on the skin, impaired taste or smell, irritability, depression, short-term memory loss, tremors, muscle weakness, headache, and malaise (tiredness). Common sources of mercury include dental fillings (amalgams; "silver" fillings contain about 50 percent mercury), fish (e.g., tuna, nonfatty freshwater fish, and swordfish), pesticides, fungicides, some vaccines (like thimerasol, a type of mercury), contact lens solution, fabric softeners, mascara (especially waterproof), some laxatives, tap water, and mercury batteries.

Even though lead has been banned as an ingredient in paint, paint is still the leading source of lead poisoning in the United States. That's because peeling lead paint can still be found on the walls of many older homes and other buildings, especially in urban areas. Children are the primary victims, not only because they tend to eat the peeling paint but also because their bodies absorb more lead per pound of body weight than adults' bodies.

Lead exposure also comes from cigarette smoke, tap water, lead-soldered pipes, glazed ceramics, pesticides, the atmosphere due to lead from coal burning, food cans with lead seams, and rain water. Exposure to lead can cause dizziness, depression, confusion, learning disabilities, gastrointestinal disorders, high blood pressure, and damage to the kidneys, liver, blood, and adrenal glands.

COMMON CHEMICALS AND OTOTOXICITY

According to the American Lung Association, the average home in the U.S. contains 45 aerosol products—paints, hobby products, personal health care products, air fresheners, cleaning agents—and many of those products contain toxic substances that can cause a variety of symptoms, including dizziness, nausea, allergic reactions, and respiratory tract irritation. Aerosol cans are not the only sources of ototoxic substances, however. To give you an idea of the many sources of chemicals that can make you dizzy and the products they are in, we've composed a representative list below.

Depending on your lifestyle and occupation, you may be exposed to more or less of these ototoxic chemicals. The severity of your reaction to any of these chemicals depends on the concentration to which you are exposed, the length of exposure time, and your body's ability to metabolize the toxin. How many of these chemicals are in your home? Note in your journal any time you experience dizziness, unsteadiness, or other symptoms when exposed to any of these substances. Also, see "What to Do About Ototoxic Substances" below.

- Benzene. A solvent commonly found in gasoline, inks, oils, paints, plastics, and rubber. It is also used during the manufacture of detergents, dyes, explosives, and pharmaceuticals. Inhalation can cause dizziness, weakness, headache, nausea, blurry vision, respiratory diseases, tremors, irregular heartbeat, and liver and kidney damage.
- Carbon monoxide. Vehicle exhaust is the most common source. Symptoms include dizziness, fatigue, headache, confusion, and nausea. Very high exposure can cause death. If you are experiencing these symptoms and have a job that typically exposes you to higher levels of exhaust, your job may be making you ill. Examples of such positions include gasoline station worker, automobile mechanic, tollbooth worker, road construction worker, bus driver, and drive-up window attendant.
- Ethylene glycol. Best known as antifreeze. Inhalation can cause dizziness, headache, nausea, and irritation of the nose, throat, and respiratory tract. Ingestion (unfortunately it has a sweet taste that attracts children) causes a "high," along with dizziness, nausea and vomiting, and sleepiness, with increasingly serious symptoms if not treated.
- Formaldehyde. Commonly found in approximately 3,000 different building products, including adhesives used in flooring,

pressed wood products, foam insulation, carpet backing, and particle board. Also found in fabric softeners, facial tissues, paper towels, waxed paper, and cigarette smoke. Symptoms associated with exposure to formaldehyde include headache, sore throat, dizziness, nausea, rash, eye irritation, and fatigue.

• Hexane. Found in gasoline, rubber cement, aerosol perfumes, paint thinner, nonmercury thermometers, and alcohol preparations. Also used in the printing, textile, furniture, and shoe making industries. Hexane is an ingredient in the glues used in roofing and in bookbinding. Short-term exposure can cause dizziness, confusion, nausea, and headache. Long-term exposure results in numbness of the hands and feet, blurry vision, muscle weakness, possible paralysis of the arms and legs, and coma.

• Imidazolidinyl urea and DMDM hydantoin. A formaldehyde-forming preservative that can cause dizziness, joint pain, headache, and insomnia. It is found in skin, body, and hair products; nail polish; and antiperspirants.

• Styrene. Found in automobile parts, carpet backing, food containers, fiberglass, insulation, rubber, plastic, and pipes. Exposure can cause depression, problems with concentration, dizziness, muscle weakness, tiredness, and nausea.

• Toluene. A by-product of the production of styrene, toluene is used in the production of gasoline, paints, paint thinner, lacquers, adhesives, nail polish, rubber, and some chemicals and is found in automobile exhaust. It can cause dizziness, nausea, tiredness, weakness, confusion, and drunken-like movements.

• Trichloroethylene. More than 90 percent of this solvent is used in the dry-cleaning business and as a solvent to remove grease from metal parts. The remainder is found in adhesives, paint removers, spot removers, and typewriter correction fluid. Exposure can cause dizziness, giddiness, loss of coordination, confusion, headache, difficulty speaking, and drowsiness.

• Xylene. One of the top 30 chemicals produced in the United States. It is a solvent used in the leather, rubber, and printing industries. Xylene is also used in paints, paint thinners, and varnishes. Exposure can cause dizziness, loss of balance, confusion, headache, and lack of muscle coordination.

WHAT TO DO ABOUT OTOTOXIC SUBSTANCES

One word—*avoidance*—is the best advice, but staying clear of ototoxic agents is not always easy. The first step is to read the product labels. The ingredient panel on the majority of health and beauty products reads like a chemical experiment. Familiarize yourself with the main ingredients in these products. The Internet is a good place to begin: type in the name of any ingredient into the "Search" box of your favorite search engine, and read up on the substance. Then take the next step. Here are a few tips:

- Switch to natural health and beauty products, such as natural soaps, shampoos, and deodorants. Many companies produce such products. (See appendix C for sources.)
- Remove toxic cleaning products from your home, including synthetic detergents, perfumed products, cleaning chemicals, and polishes. Use natural products which are safer, better for the environment, and less costly. These include vinegar, lemons, baking soda, and borax.
- When working on your house or hobbies, use nontoxic stains, paints, and varnishes.
- Avoid dry cleaning.
- Do not smoke, and do not allow smokers in your home or work space.
- Use a quality water filter. A reverse osmosis–carbon block filter can remove synthetic chemicals and heavy metals from your water. Suppliers of water filters can be found in appendix C.
- Surround yourself with pollution-reducing plants. Certain plants, including English ivy, Chinese evergreen, corn plant,

dieffenbachia, spider plant, wandering jew, and bamboo palm, remove chemicals such as benzene, formaldehyde, and trichloroethylene from the air.

- Use nontoxic methods of pest control for your lawn and home. Boric acid, garlic sprays, diatomaceous earth, insecticidal soaps, pheromone traps, beneficial insects, and other methods can be effective. Check with organic gardening organizations and websites for more information (see appendix C).

Alcohol, Caffeine, and Nicotine

Because they aren't illegal and are in fact widely used and advertised, we usually don't think of alcohol, caffeine, and nicotine as drugs. Yet these three popular chemicals can have serious negative effects on the body. Here we concern ourselves with their impact on the vestibular system.

ALCOHOL

In small amounts and when taken infrequently, alcohol can be relatively harmless for most people. Unfortunately, excessive and abusive use of alcohol is common among people of all ages. It is becoming increasingly more common among older adults, when a combination of alcohol abuse and a decline in muscle strength, flexibility, and reflexes can result in great loss of balance, falls, and fractures.

Common signs and symptoms of alcohol abuse include difficulty with balance and walking, muscle weakness, memory problems, poor nutrition, high blood pressure, liver disease, low blood sugar, osteoporosis, gastrointestinal problems, arrhythmias, and reproductive problems. Prolonged use of alcohol can also have a significant impact on the nervous system (see "Neuropathy" in chapter 8). Damage to the nervous system often has an early start: it's estimated that up to 40 percent of all men in their teens and twenties have had an alcoholic blackout.

Alcoholism can also cause a condition called Wernicke's syndrome, in which people experience poor balance, problems with walking, nystagmus (abnormal eye movements), double vision, and mental confusion. Wernicke's syndrome is associated with a severe deficiency of the B vitamin thiamin. Alcohol also appears to increase the body's need for B vitamins while interfering with the body's ability to absorb thiamin. Because thiamin plays a key role in providing energy for brain cells, a deficiency of it leads to the symptoms mentioned. Treatment with thiamin can help improve problems with balance and walking, but about 50 percent of people continue to have some difficulties.

CAFFEINE

We like to think of coffee, tea, and colas as refreshing, tasty beverages, but we also need to remember that, in most cases, they contain caffeine, a chemical that speeds up heart rate and breathing and raises the level of stress hormones in the body. For people who drink too much of caffeinated beverages—and "too much" varies by individual—the result is often dizziness, jitters, headache, insomnia, and restlessness. You may get the same symptoms from eating chocolate, which contains theobromine and theophylline—ingredients that are similar to caffeine. Many over-the-counter and prescription medications also contain caffeine.

If caffeine is causing or contributing to your feelings of dizziness and lightheadedness, it's probably time to eliminate it from your diet. Hints on how to do so, plus a list of the caffeine content of various beverages and other products, are in chapter 13.

NICOTINE

Faster than a speeding bullet, or, more appropriately, faster than a heroin injection takes effect, that's how long it takes for nicotine to reach the brain. When you inhale smoke into your lungs, the nicotine is picked up by the bloodstream, and the heart pumps the blood to the brain. All of this takes just seven seconds, and the result is a nicotine "high."

Nicotine makes the heart beat faster, which increases the breathing rate. Blood vessels become narrow, which slows down blood flow and thus raises blood pressure. These effects on the cardiovascular system can cause lightheadedness and dizziness in many smokers.

If you smoke excessively (or used to), you may have developed nicotine poisoning. This condition is characterized by dizziness, numbness in the fingers, nausea, vomiting, weakness, and gastrointestinal distress. These symptoms are also characteristic of people who smoke while using smoking-cessation products, such as a nicotine patch or nicotine gum. Children who ingest nicotine gum also can experience these symptoms, as well as unconsciousness.

Stopping smoking can also make you dizzy. Symptoms of nicotine withdrawal can include dizziness, anxiety, depression, fatigue, difficulty sleeping, and problems with concentration. Fortunately, these symptoms are temporary and part of the detoxification process the body goes through when ridding itself of a poison like nicotine.

Bottom Line

Thousands of products and substances that you come into contact with daily in your life and environment have the potential to cause dizziness and balance problems. It's up to you to do your best to recognize these toxins and to avoid them when possible. Take a look around your home, garden, and workplace to see which of these toxins are present and which ones you can eliminate and replace with safer items or less toxic approaches. Although it may seem that exposure to a small amount of exhaust or chemicals from carpeting or secondhand smoke or aerosol sprays individually couldn't have much effect on your nervous system, remember that you are likely being exposed to many "small amounts" every day, and these can add up to a significant impact on your health and sense of balance.

10

In Your Head: Psychological Dizziness

For many people, depression, anxiety, or phobia is the cause of their dizziness or related symptoms. Don't think that because the cause is "in your head" that it isn't real. Balance problems associated with psychological disorders are just as uncomfortable and debilitating as those caused by physical disorders.

Although you may not think dizziness is a common characteristic of psychological disorders, about 10 percent of vestibular symptoms have psychological origins. In fact, dizziness is the second most common symptom reported by individuals who have panic disorder. Panic disorder is also common among people who undergo vestibular testing. Another interesting fact is that the symptoms experienced during an episode of vertigo (excessive sweating, rapid heartbeat, and nausea) also often occur during a panic attack. And, as you'll see below, dizziness is commonly a part of depression.

These associations suggest that psychological conditions are a risk factor for dizziness and should be considered seriously by patients and doctors during an examination. Let's look at a few of those conditions now.

Anxiety and Panic Disorders

Shortness of breath, dizziness, feeling like you're going to faint, and heart palpitations—if you suffer with anxiety, you probably recognize these symptoms. They, along with sweating, chills, tremors, chest pain, numbness or tingling in the extremities, and a lump in the throat are common occurrences among people who suffer with anxiety disorders, and those are more than 19 million Americans.

One common symptom of anxiety is hyperventilation, or breathing harder and faster than normal. Hyperventilation causes the amount of carbon dioxide in your blood to drop, which results in lightheadedness, faintness, and tingling and numbness in the fingers and toes.

Sudden, intense episodes of overwhelming anxiety or panic, commonly referred to as panic or anxiety attacks, affect a percentage of people who live with anxiety. Dizziness and fainting are often part of these attacks, which lead some people to believe they are having a heart attack or that they are losing their mind. This fear only adds to an already frightening experience. If you have had anxiety attacks, explain the circumstances as clearly as possible to your health-care providers so they can make a more accurate assessment of your condition.

TREATMENT

Anxiety and panic disorders are treated with psychotherapy, cognitive behavioral therapies, and medications (sedatives such as diazepam or alprazolam and/or beta blockers). If you have an anxiety disorder and a vestibular problem, vestibular rehabilitation may be added as part of your treatment plan. If you take medications, here's what to expect.

- Sedatives. Two commonly used sedatives are alprazolam (Xanax) and diazepam (Valium; also Diastat, Diazepam Intensol, and Dizac). Alprazolam relieves anxiety and the dizziness that can accompany it. Diazepam is effective against vertigo. Both drugs have drowsiness as a common side effect, and both are addictive.
- Beta-blockers (atenolol [Tenomin], metaprolol [Lopressor], propranolol [Inderal], nadolol [Congard], and timolol [Blocadren]). Limit the ability of blood vessels to overdilate (expand). Side effects can include drowsiness, dry mouth, eyes, and skin; cold hands and feet; and dizziness.

BRANDY'S STORY

For more than three years, Brandy, a 40-year-old administrative assistant, had been experiencing mild but constant lightheadedness and disequilibrium. Her symptoms were usually not serious enough to prevent her from working, but she said she just never "felt right."

Brandy also noted that when she was in certain situations, such as driving on winding roads or going into supermarkets, shopping malls, or other crowded environments, her symptoms grew worse. On those occasions, her dizziness was usually accompanied by tingling in her hands and feet. Her remedy had been to avoid these circumstances whenever possible.

Brandy came to see me on a referral from her primary care physician, whose preliminary physical examination had revealed nothing unusual. She said she never experienced any hearing loss or ringing in her ears. My neurological examination of Brandy showed some abnormal eye movements of which she was not aware and which suggested an anxiety disorder. Her electronystagmography and posturography tests were normal.

On the basis of her symptoms, the presence of abnormal eye movements, and the lack of any signs of a vestibular disease, I diagnosed Brandy as having an anxiety disorder. I recommended that she undergo behavioral therapy and consider stress management (e.g., meditation, visualization, and biofeedback) and also prescribed a low dose of a sedative (diazepam).

After two months of treatment, Brandy reported that her symptoms had vastly improved. She continues to take a low dose of diazepam and practices meditation daily.

Depression

We hear a lot of talk about how to identify the symptoms of depression. Typically we're told that feeling sad all or most of the time, losing interest in things and people that once pleased us, and experiencing reduced sexual desire, among other factors, are all indications of depression.

However, dizziness, lightheadedness, and vertigo can be common indications of depression as well. In fact, some people who are depressed display dizziness rather than the typical symptoms. This type of depression is called *masked depression* and can be difficult to diagnose because the people affected usually function well in their lives, or at least appear to do so. Although they don't complain about their low mood, they often have physical symptoms of depression, such as dizziness, vertigo, aches and pains, palpitations, gastrointestinal problems, and headache.

The fact that masked depression exists is yet another reason why it is important to tell your health-care providers about *all* the symptoms you are experiencing. One way to help you do this is to keep a diary of your symptoms: when they occur, whether there were any precipitating events, and how long the symptoms last.

Treatment of depression includes psychotherapy, stress management, medication, or a combination of these approaches. Once individuals are able to successfully identify and manage their depression, the symptoms disappear.

Phobias

If the sight of a spider or dog fills you with dread, if you panic at the thought of boarding a plane, or if you are terrified of elevators, you likely have a phobia. A phobia is a type of anxiety disorder that is characterized by an overwhelming feeling of terror, dread, or panic that occurs when someone thinks about, sees, or comes face to face with a specific situation, object, or activity. About 11.5 million Americans (8 percent of adults) have at least one phobia.

Some experts have identified a condition called phobic vertigo in which people experience a sudden, frightening feeling that they are going to fall, even if they are sitting down. The dizziness may be mild and not too disruptive, or a vertigo attack may occur and actually cause a fall. These dizziness and vertigo episodes are typically associated with emotional stress. If you experience such attacks, it's important for you to keep a diary of the events surrounding them so you and your doctor can work out a way for you to manage and eliminate these experiences.

Acrophobia—fear of heights—occurs when physiological height vertigo (see chapter 5) triggers an involuntary phobic reaction of intense fear, anxiety, and even hysteria. Several studies have concluded that some people develop a fear of heights because they are highly susceptible to motion sickness when they are in a height situation and are frightened by these symptoms of the motion sickness.

The psychological treatment of phobias may include behavioral therapy, desensitization (repeated, therapist-guided exposure to the object or situation until the phobic response disappears), and medication, such as the sedatives alprazolam (Xanax) and diazepam (Valium), among others (see "Anxiety and Panic Disorders" above).

Somatization

People who have unexplained dizziness often meet the criteria for a psychological condition called somatization, a medical term for what was at one time referred to as hypochondria or hysteria. Dizziness is one of the most commonly reported complaints that cause individuals to seek a doctor's advice. Others include muscle weakness, fatigue, headache, incoordination, confusion, depression, and/or anxiety.

Typically, individuals with somatization disorder experience many different symptoms that cause them to make repeated visits to their doctors and to try various medications. They undergo numerous tests and examinations, yet doctors can find no physical reasons for their complaints. This doesn't mean these people don't really experience their symptoms. Their pain and discomfort are physical expressions of unconsciously held psychological conflicts, anxieties, emotional stresses, or unresolved issues. In fact, up to 50 percent of people with somatization disorder also have an anxiety disorder, and up to 60 percent suffer with some type of depression.

A diagnosis of somatization is usually one of elimination: health-care practitioners make the diagnosis after they get negative results on tests and examinations and can find no physical cause for a patient's symptoms. People who have somatization disorder typically will not acknowledge that they have a psychological condition when they are told of the diagnosis, so treatment is often a problem. If you have a loved one who is displaying the characteristic signs and symptoms of somatization, a combination of emotional support from you, a caring physician, and psychotherapy can help in alleviating the symptoms of dizziness and other physical problems.

Bottom Line

Depression and other psychological disorders are very common, and it's important that you and your doctors recognize that dizziness and disequilibrium are frequently part of these disorders. Similar to the physiological conditions we've discussed in the previous chapters, treatment of the underlying illness, be it depression, anxiety, or phobia, is necessary to eliminate the symptoms of dizziness and/or disequilibrium. Often, a combination treatment approach of behavioral or cognitive therapy along with medication and stress management techniques is effective.

11

What to Expect If You Need
Special Tests

If you've turned to this chapter, you've probably been referred to
a specialist to undergo further testing. The mere thought of
having to take "special tests" may cause you some stress or concern, but we want to let you know you have no need to worry.
These tests are not painful, although a few of them may cause
you some mild discomfort. In the end, however, they can provide
a wealth of information to your doctors and a more direct path to
effective treatment for you.

We believe that before you undergo any specialized testing,
it's best to understand why the test is necessary, what the doctor
or technician will be doing, and what the results will reveal. The
following explanations can increase your understanding of these
procedures and prepare you for when you talk to your doctor
about them.

Will you need to undergo a lot of tests? Probably not. You see a lot of tests listed here (and there are many more) because there are dozens from which your doctors may choose. Because we have no way of knowing which one or more they will select for you, we have listed some of the most common ones.

I always encourage my patients to provide as many details as they can on their medical history and dizziness questionnaire, because these two tools, along with the results of a thorough physical examination, can give invaluable information for making a diagnosis. However, specialized tests often provide the "aha" factor, the answer you and your doctors have been looking for.

Electronystagmography Testing

Electronystagmography (ENG) testing consists of a battery of six tests that evaluate the relationship between your inner ear and your eyes. The tests have been in use since the 1940s, but over the years their levels of accuracy and sophistication have improved greatly. The information doctors gather from these tests, which are discussed below, can help them determine whether your dizziness or vertigo is caused by a problem in the inner ear (vestibular system) or in the central nervous system. Doctors order an ENG because of suspicions raised by the information gathered from your medical history, dizziness questionnaire, and physical examination. It is one of the most common special tests given to people who suffer with vertigo, dizziness, or disequilibrium.

When you move your head, your inner ears are stimulated, and signals are sent to your eye muscles via your nervous system. This function is known as the vestibulo-ocular (inner ear–visual) reflex (VOR). When both your vestibular and visual systems are operating correctly, your vision remains clear when you move your head. If something is wrong, you can experience dizziness or vertigo.

Electronystagmography is designed to help find the problem. It is a painless procedure that involves attaching electrodes to the skin on the face and around the eyes. The electrodes measure involuntary eye movements (nystagmus; movements may be side to side, up and down, or rotating) and how they relate to the vestibular system during various tests that stimulate the inner ear. Your doctor may choose to do several or all of the tests explained below.

In preparation for these tests, your doctor will ask you to refrain from taking antihistamines, antidepressants, any medications for dizziness, or other drugs. You will likely be allowed to continue to take drugs for heart disease or blood pressure; talk to your doctor about these medications.

Here are the six tests that are included under the general title electronystagmography.

CALORIC TESTING

When used in this sense, caloric refers to temperature and has nothing to do with food. In this test, warm and cold water or air or both are placed into the ear canals individually. The introduction of warm and cold stimuli causes the endolymph fluid in the inner ear to either expand or contract, respectively. This slight movement fools the vestibular system into thinking that the head is moving. It also triggers involuntary eye movements, which the doctor or technician record with the electrodes placed near the eyes. If electrodes are not used, that is, if the equipment is not available or a doctor is performing the test during a home or nursing home visit, he or she will observe and note the movements.

If the eye movements are up and down, they suggest a problem in brain function. The speed at which the eyes move is recorded, because it can help reveal the extent of function in the vestibular system. The ears are typically tested one at a time, using either the warm or cold stimulus, and then a few minutes are allowed to pass before the next ear or stimulus is tested. In some cases, however, doctors test both ears at the same time.

You may experience some slight discomfort during this test, depending on the temperature of the water or air (the colder the stimulus, the greater risk for discomfort or pain) and the speed at which the stimulus is introduced into the ear. Some people report mild dizziness or nausea, while others experience vertigo or ear pain. Fortunately, these symptoms disappear quickly, and they do provide the doctor with important information.

GAZE TEST

While sitting with your head still, you will be asked to look at various dots or lights that will be placed 20 to 30 degrees to your left and right. During this time, the electrodes will record your eye movements. As with the caloric test, if nystagmus is from side to side, it suggests a problem in the vestibular system.

Doctors use this test to detect any nystagmus they may not have noted during their observations.

SACCADE AND CALIBRATION TEST

You will be asked to look alternately at two objects or lights that have been placed a specific distance apart. The electrodes will measure the speed at which your eyes move. If your eyes move more slowly than the acceptable range, certain problems are indicated. For example, slow movements suggest that your brain has a problem controlling your eyes, especially if the movement follows a certain pattern. People who have Parkinson's disease, Huntington's disease, multiple sclerosis, or a lesion on their cerebellum may have slow eye movement on this test. Abnormally slow movement may also be a sign of a vision problem.

OPTOKINETIC TEST

We talked about the optokinetic system and its role in balance in chapter 1. Here's the test to see how it's functioning.

As you sit in a chair, your eye movements will be recorded while you look at a pattern of stripes or other large, simple objects as they move at a constant speed horizontally back and forth in front of you. In some facilities, the chair moves rather than the pattern. In either case, the effect is the same: to elicit a response from the optokinetic reflex, which is the reflex that helps you keep your eyes fixed on a target when your head moves. Results of this test may reveal which ear has the damage that is causing or contributing to your dizziness or vertigo.

SMOOTH PURSUIT TEST

In this test, reminiscent of a session with a hypnotist, the tester will swing a pendulum or pencil across your field of vision as you sit with your head perfectly still. The electrodes will record your eye movements, which should be smooth. If, however, they are erratic, that may be the result of your having taken certain medications (e.g., anticonvulsants, lithium, some antihistamines, or alcohol), all of which hinder the function of the brain stem and cerebellum, or it may indicate a lesion on the brain. This test is not always accurate in people who are elderly or who have poor visual acuity, as they generally will have erratic eye movements.

DIX-HALLPIKE MANEUVER

To ensure that your eye movements are in response to the positions you are placed in and not to the objects in the room, you will be asked to wear Frenzel goggles. These special magnifying glasses cause everything you see to be very blurry, but they also allow the doctor to easily observe your eye movements.

From a sitting position on an examining table or bed, you will lie down with your head hanging off the edge of the table or bed. Your doctor will support your head. You will remain with your head hanging for about 20 seconds; then you'll be helped up to a sitting position. The doctor will repeat this process several times, holding your head between his or her hands while placing your head in a different position each time. The doctor will be looking for any nystagmus, and if it occurs, it can provide clues as to the cause of your dizziness.

Audiogram

It is not uncommon for people who suffer with dizziness or a balance disorder to also have some degree of hearing loss or other hearing problem. After all, the cochlea, which contains the organ of hearing (the spiral organ of Corti), resides in the inner ear along with all the balance structures. If something goes wrong with your hearing, damage to the inner ear may accompany it.

Even if you have no hearing complaints, an audiogram may be requested to evaluate the integrity of your inner ear function. It sometimes reveals changes in hearing at certain frequencies of which you may not be aware, or some asymmetries between the ears. Since the inner ears are deeply seated inside the head and are not visible to the examiner, testing their function is a crucial way to determine their health status. An audiogram for the ear is what the electrocardiogram (EKG) is for the heart.

Hearing tests, called audiograms, are usually done by hearing specialists, or audiologists. These painless procedures are conducted while you sit in a soundproof room or booth that has at least one two-way window. You will wear earphones and be instructed by an audiologist, who sits outside the booth, to give signals when you hear certain words or sounds.

Audiograms can distinguish between two different types of hearing problems: conductive hearing loss and sensorineural hearing loss. Conductive hearing loss occurs when there's a problem with the transmission of signals from the outer ear through the eardrum into the inner ear. Sensorineural hearing loss usually is the result of damaged hair cells in the cochlea or an abnormality of the auditory nerve. Such problems can be caused by infections, trauma, immune-related disorders, degenerative processes of aging, exposure to excessively loud noise, or taking certain medications, or they may be hereditary or congenital.

An acoustic neuroma, a type of noncancerous tumor (see chapter 5), is one cause of sensorineural hearing loss. This tumor is also associated with ringing in the ears, imbalance, and an unsteady gait.

Auditory Brain Stem Response Test

The auditory brain stem response test, also known as the brain stem evoked response audiometry, is another type of hearing test in which you wear earphones. This time, however, the doctor evaluates electric activity by monitoring your brain waves as you listen to clicking sounds. The electrodes attached to your scalp record your brain waves on a computer screen, which indicates the amount of time it takes for the nerves to transmit the signals from your ear to your brain. If there is an abnormality somewhere along the nerve pathways, the graph will show a delay as well as indicate where the problem is located.

Electrocochleography

This test measures the electric responses that occur within the cochlea and the eighth nerve when they are stimulated. This measurement can be gathered by placing an electrode as close as possible to the cochlea. The electrode is usually placed deep inside the ear canal. In some cases, the electrode must be placed surgically through the eardrum onto the surface of the inner ear.

Electrocochleography is most often used to diagnose or monitor Ménière's disease (see chapter 4). The reason is that this test can show whether there is an increase in endolymph pressure, which is a sign of endolymphatic hydrops and a definite sign of Ménière's disease.

Rotary Chair Test

This is a test many people think of when they hear they need to undergo balance testing. Rotational chair testing has been used for decades to determine the integrity of the vestibular system, specifically to measure the vestibulo-ocular reflex. Unlike the rotary chair test of prior decades, today's procedure is computerized.

Once electrodes have been placed on your head, the test chair will begin to tilt back and forth, and then rotate more and more rapidly. The electrodes record your eye movements in relation to the speed of the chair. Because this test is typically conducted in the dark, your eyes will not be distracted by other objects in the room. If the test shows less eye movement when your head is turned to one side or the other, it reveals a loss or asymmetry in vestibular function.

Fistula Test

If your otologist and audiologist suspect your dizziness may be a symptom of a perilymphatic fistula (see below), this test will be done. It is based on the principle that changes in air pressure in the ear can trigger dizziness.

Like the ENG tests, this test involves placing electrodes on your face so your responses can be recorded. The audiologist will then place a probe into your ear and change the air pressure, both up and down, to see if there are any changes in nystagmic activity or in the level of dizziness you experience. The results of this test, along with others, are used to make a diagnosis of perilymphatic fistula.

Computerized Platform Posturography

This test allows your doctor to determine how much motor control and balance you can maintain in different environmental conditions. Computerized platform posturography gathers information about the integrity of the signals your brain receives from your proprioceptive system—your muscles, joints, skin, and tendons—and how they interact with the signals from your inner ears and eyes.

This test differs from all the others in that you will wear a safety harness. This is merely a precaution to prevent you from falling in case you lose your balance during the procedure. The test involves standing on a computer-controlled platform that is located just inside a three-sided box. The sides of the box are covered with a scene, such as a forest or beach, or colors. The technician will cause the platform to tilt. Pressure gauges under the platform record your shifting weight and the amount you sway.

Computerized platform posturography allows the doctor to test the reliability of your proprioceptive, visual, and vestibular systems. When the technician moves the platform, the sensors in your ankles and feet transmit signals to your brain. Because the platform's position changes, you depend more on your vision to help you maintain balance. If you lose your balance, the computer records information about the signals. If the technician were to blindfold you and then tilt the platform, you would have to depend on your vestibular system to keep your balance. If you lose your balance once your vision is removed and your proprioceptive system is being challenged, this indicates your balance problem may be in your vestibular system.

This test is not performed as often as some of the others because it uses very expensive equipment and it duplicates information that can be gathered from other, less costly tests. However, it can be very helpful for examining patients who are difficult to diagnose.

Scans

Sometimes doctors order scans—computerized tomography (CT) scans or magnetic resonance imaging (MRI) scans—to find the source of a balance disorder. A CT scan is a three-dimensional x-ray that can detect abnormalities in the bony structures of the ear and surrounding areas. An MRI uses a magnetic field and radio waves to image body parts. It can be used to scan the brain to look for damage from stroke, tumors, or other abnormalities or to image the inner ear to locate a possible tumor.

Bottom Line

The use of specialized tests can help your doctors zero in on the cause of your dizziness, vertigo, and/or disequilibrium problems. The tests covered in this chapter are among the most common ones given; however, there are others that your doctors may order for you. Whether you are asked to undergo some of the tests in this chapter or others not listed, we encourage you to be an informed, involved health-care consumer.

- Ask questions of your doctors about your condition and any tests you've been asked to take. If you don't understand the answers, ask again. If they are reluctant to answer you, ask if there is someone else who can help you or find another doctor.
- Become more informed. Don't just read this book; explore the Suggested Reading as well. Talk to other people who have balance problems, and keep track of the latest research in the field. You can contact some of the organizations listed in the appendix and ask to be on their mailing list, or join an email newsletter service that will keep you posted on new developments.

Dizziness, vertigo, and disequilibrium are symptoms, not diseases. Literally dozens of medical conditions or other circumstances can be behind these symptoms. Arriving at a diagnosis is not always an easy task, and misdiagnosis is a possibility if the investigation is not thorough. Therefore, work along with your doctors so you'll have a better chance of quickly uncovering the root of your problems and moving on toward a solution.

PART III

STOP THE WORLD: TREATING BALANCE DISORDERS

You've reached the part of the book in which we talk about solutions: how to manage, treat, and eliminate dizziness, vertigo, disequilibrium, and their associated symptoms. You've seen that dizziness and balance disorders can be difficult to diagnose, so it's no surprise that treating them can take a multifaceted approach. We've broken down those approaches into four areas: (1) vestibular rehabilitation therapy and other physical therapies, (2) diet, (3) surgery, and (4) complementary approaches. (When applicable, use of medications has been discussed for individual disorders under "Treatment" in chapters 4 through 10. A summary of medications can be found in appendix A.)

In my practice, I recommend that my patients begin with the least invasive approaches: dietary changes, minimal medications as needed, maneuvers if the diagnosis is BPPV, and, only if absolutely necessary, a surgical procedure. Naturally, you should discuss all your therapeutic options with your health-care providers.

Some of the solutions discussed in the four chapters that follow will eliminate your dizziness or imbalance problems. Others will greatly improve your quality of life, even though some light-headedness or unsteadiness may persist. Some treatment approaches will produce results almost immediately; others may take weeks or months before progress is apparent.

The good news is that there are many options open to you and those you love who may be living with a balance problem. You can use the information in these chapters as a starting point of discussion with your doctors about treatment for you.

Basically there are two approaches to healing:

• If the cause of your dizziness, vertigo, and/or disequilibrium is an underlying disease or condition, you need to treat that disease. Depending on the ailment, you may be working primarily with your primary care physician, cardiologist, endocrinologist, neurologist, or psychiatrist, for example. Often, effective treatment of the underlying condition will eliminate or at least reduce your symptoms. Vestibular rehabilitation therapy and/or complementary medicine remedies may supplement your treatment approach, depending on the underlying condition.

• If your symptoms are the result of a vestibular problem, you'll likely be treated primarily by an otolaryngologist or neurotologist and, depending on the diagnosis, balance rehabilitation therapists, and perhaps various complementary medicine practitioners.

If you've been living with a balance disorder, you know how frustrating it can be. It's time for that frustration to end and for healing to begin. Some of the approaches discussed in these chapters can be done by you entirely without a physician. However, we recommend that you consult with your doctor(s) before starting any treatment, including dietary and complementary therapies.

12

Vestibular Rehabilitation and Other Physical Therapies

At this very moment, you possess one of the most important tools you can use to conquer your dizziness or balance problem. We're not talking about pills or low-salt diets or decaffeinated coffee; we're talking about your body's natural and inherent ability to heal itself.

This natural healing power takes many forms, and one of the most interesting features is the plasticity of the central nervous system. That is, the brain has the ability to be shaped and molded, to compensate for damage to the vestibular system and for mismatched signals that come to it from the peripheral nervous system because of aging, vestibular disorders, visual problems, sensory disorders, prolonged use of vestibular suppressant medications, or other conditions. If your left inner ear says up but your right inner ear says down, what happens? The brain compensates. If your eyes tell you you're seeing a room that is horizontal but your feet sense that the floor is slanted? The brain compensates. And it is because this natural wonder of compensation exists that vestibular rehabilitation therapy works.

Although the concept of vestibular rehabilitation therapy was introduced several decades ago, in recent years it has been built on, been modified, and as a result, become more effective. More and more doctors are realizing the power of this approach, and so more patients are being referred to facilities for this treatment.

In this chapter we discuss many of the facets of the therapeutic approach and how it can not only reduce or eliminate your dizziness, vertigo, and disequilibrium but also improve your strength, flexibility, and posture. We also offer some exercises you can do at home (with the permission of your doctor, of course), complete with instructions, and without the need for any equipment.

We also talk about two other special types of physical therapies that have proven themselves to be very effective for people with balance problems. One is a group of three very similar maneuvers used to treat benign paroxysmal positional vertigo. These techniques are so successful, as many as 80 percent of patients who undergo these quick, simple, and painless procedures are free of BPPV after only one treatment.

The other therapy is tai chi, an ancient Chinese exercise technique that is helpful if you have balance problems. Tai chi is especially beneficial for older adults, as it is not strenuous yet can build balance, strength, and flexibility, as well as self-confidence as all these things improve.

Is Vestibular Rehabilitation Therapy for You?

If you're sitting at home reading this book and have been experiencing periodic vertigo episodes, can you simply drive to your nearest vestibular rehabilitation center and sign up? Not exactly. As you've seen in earlier chapters, dizziness, vertigo, and disequilibrium can be caused by or associated with dozens of conditions—conditions that are not always easy to diagnose—and the cause of your balance problems will dictate the treatment approach. Thus an accurate diagnosis is essential before treatment is initiated.

Most people, but not all, who have a problem with dizziness or balance can benefit from vestibular rehabilitation therapy. Generally, the people who benefit most from this approach fall into these categories:

• People who have an inner ear disorder that is being treated with diet and/or medication but who still have some bothersome dizziness or balance problems that can be more quickly remedied with rehabilitation. Such conditions may include labyrinthitis, vestibular neuronitis, Ménière's disease, head injury, chronic ear infection, or otosclerosis.

• People who have age-related difficulties with balance. Vestibular rehabilitation therapy can be instrumental in helping elderly individuals maintain strength and balance so they can retain independence and in teaching them how to prevent falls.

• People who have tried drugs designed to suppress vertigo and its associated symptoms (see appendix A) and have had little or no relief. Many of these medications have side effects that can limit people's ability to function optimally, and they also hinder the brain's ability to compensate.

• People who have secondary symptoms associated with dizziness or disequilibrium, such as muscle weakness, limited range of motion, visual problems, and joint pain that affect their coordination and balance. This category may include people who have arthritis, multiple sclerosis, cataracts, stroke, diabetes, or peripheral neuropathy. They can benefit from strengthening exercises, vision exercises, and other assistance not directly related to balance.

• People who have undergone surgery that has instantaneously eliminated their balance function (e.g., labyrinthectomy or vestibular nerve section; see chapter 14). These procedures are typically performed on individuals who have debilitating Ménière's disease. Balance rehabilitation can accelerate the rate of their recovery.

• People who have dizziness and/or disequilibrium associated with a psychological condition. Vestibular rehabilitation therapy can help them feel more secure about their balance and ease anxiety, which often fuels balance disorders.

Before you can enter a vestibular rehabilitation therapy program, in most states you will need to be referred by a physician, usually an otolaryngologist, neurologist, or neurotologist. He or she provides the rehabilitation team with information about your specific diagnosis, past medical history, medications you are taking, and any test results. Then you will be ready for a thorough evaluation by a physical therapist.

What Is Vestibular Rehabilitation Therapy?

Vestibular rehabilitation therapy consists of various exercises and maneuvers that are designed to help the brain compensate for the conditions that are causing dizziness, vertigo, and disequilibrium. The goal of therapy is to eliminate or significantly reduce symptoms and to improve:

• Equilibrium
• Mobility
• Overall physical condition and activity level, including strength, flexibility, and range of motion
• Safety

The different activities are tailored to the specific needs and limitations of individual patients, and no two therapy plans are alike.

Vestibular rehabilitation therapy can be used instead of or in addition to medication and/or surgery and/or dietary approaches and/or complementary techniques. It can make a dramatic difference in the lives of people who are living with dizziness, vertigo, and disequilibrium. People who once were afraid to leave their homes because they never knew when they would experience a vertigo episode or suffer a fall have regained their independence once they participated in vestibular rehabilitation therapy. Men and women who had given up their careers, schooling, travel plans, and social lives have been able to return to their former lifestyles.

Depending on the severity of your condition, you will need to attend one to two sessions a week at a vestibular rehabilitation facility, where you will work with professionals who have chosen the exercises and maneuvers especially for your needs. The exercises may focus on eye, head, posture, and balance movements that help recondition your balance system and compensate for any loss or imbalance you have experienced. You may also work on building strength in your lower limbs to help improve your balance.

One beauty of vestibular rehabilitation therapy is that much of it can be done at home. From the beginning of your therapy, you will be given a detailed plan of exercises to do at home to supplement the work you do at the facility. Your therapy will be successful only if *you* do the work.

WHAT TO EXPECT FROM VESTIBULAR REHABILITATION THERAPY

Depending on your condition, rehabilitation therapy can be completed in as little as four weeks, but may last eight or more. Six to eight weeks is the norm for people who have a problem with one ear only (unilateral loss). If you are affected in both ears (bilateral loss), such as when you have bilateral Ménière's disease or you have undergone a destructive surgical technique (e.g., labyrinthectomy), you will need a longer treatment program. Your therapist will reassess your progress every week or so and make adjustments to your therapy as needed. Once you're "graduated" from rehabilitation therapy, you may need or want to continue to do your home exercises.

Regardless of whether you have experienced loss of balance in one or both ears, you should know that during your first few therapy sessions, your symptoms may worsen temporarily before they get better. Don't get discouraged; it takes more than one session to retrain your brain. In fact, the main premise of vestibular rehabilitation therapy is to simulate conditions that are known to make you dizzy in order to help you stop getting dizzy. Although this sounds like a crazy way to treat dizziness, this approach works.

Also consider that factors such as your age, the presence of any other physical problems or emotional disorders, and your compliance with the program will have an impact on how well you respond to therapy. It's important that you do your home exercises every day, as prescribed by your therapist, in order to get the maximum benefit from your program.

COMPONENTS OF VESTIBULAR REHABILITATION THERAPY

A comprehensive vestibular rehabilitation therapy program consists of the following components. Many of the exercises that make up a vestibular rehabilitation program fall into more than one category, so these classifications are not hard-and-fast. A balance exercise, for example, may also incorporate gait or vestibular stimulation features, and proprioception tasks often incorporate balance components.

• Strengthening exercises. May include working with light weights or simple exercises to strengthen the lower extremities. Strengthening exercises are especially important for people who have a condition characterized by muscle weakness, people with arthritis, people who have suffered a stroke, or older adults who have age-related muscle weakness.

• Safety awareness and patient education. Especially critical for older adults who are prone to falls and fractures. Some people are referred to vestibular rehabilitation even though they don't have a vestibular disorder, but they have trouble with balance because of poor eyesight, arthritis, or muscle weakness. These individuals may work with an occupational therapist (see below) as well as learn various exercises. Patients are instructed on ways to make their homes safe (see box, p. 202), how to maneuver safely in different environments, and how to use different devices, such as canes, walkers, and grip bars.

• Balance, gait, and postural exercises. Designed to retrain your balance system, improve muscle coordination and responses, and improve your gait and posture.

• Vestibular stimulation. Movements that stimulate the semicircular canals and nerves of the inner ear to help you retrain your balance system. Exercises may include those which ask you to move your head in specific ways or even to perform simple ballet movements. The exercises are based on the concept that by repeatedly exposing yourself to specific stimuli that cause dizziness or vertigo *for you specifically,* your brain will reduce and then eliminate the vertigo. You may be asked to keep a daily diary that documents how often you do the exercises and how you respond to them.

• Proprioception tasks. Movements that challenge your sensory input, such as walking on soft surfaces (e.g., pillows or foam rubber) or uneven terrain such as sand or grass.

• Sensory integration. Exercises that improve your ability to interpret and integrate sensory input and to compensate when signals from another system have been lost or compromised.

YOUR VESTIBULAR REHABILITATION TEAM

The various professionals involved in your therapy will decide which areas need to be addressed, on the basis of the recommendations of your neurotologist or other referring physician. Together these professionals are a team and may include the following individuals. (Not everyone who participates in vestibular rehabilitation therapy utilizes all of these team members.):

• Physical therapists. Their job is to evaluate your condition, consult with other team members, and devise a treatment plan especially for you. They will then demonstrate and help you with the exercises that you will do at the facility and those you will do at home. These can include strengthening or gait exercises, hand-to-eye coordination exercises, tasks to improve proprioceptive abilities, and balance and postural exercises.

• Occupational therapists. The task of occupational therapists is to help individuals learn alternative ways to regain or achieve independence in everyday activities. They are especially helpful for elderly people who have lost some of their strength, vision, or other abilities and may not be able to return to their earlier level of functioning. Occupational therapists may recommend special lighting or the installation of handrails in certain areas of the home or of other equipment that will help people maintain balance.

• Vision specialists. If you are experiencing vision problems that are affecting your balance or causing dizziness, vision specialists can recommend appropriate glasses or lenses that may help. They can also teach you special exercises that can help your brain compensate for the mismatch of visual stimuli going to your brain.

• Audiologists. Their role is to perform hearing evaluations and conduct hearing and balance diagnostic tests described earlier. Because hearing loss is frequently part of a vestibular problem, hearing aids may become necessary.

• Nutritionists/dietitians. Nutritional guidance concerning a low-salt diet, eliminating caffeine, and supplementation with various nutrients can be offered by qualified nutritionists or dietitians as needed.

• Mental health professionals. Dizziness and balance problems are more than physical conditions; they can cause fear, anxiety, depression, and embarrassment. Regaining emotional and mental health is just as important as restoring physical well-being, so the assistance of social workers, psychologists, or psychiatrists may be needed. They may also recommend that you join a support group for people who have Ménière's disease or other balance problems.

Evaluation Before Entering Rehabilitation Therapy

Even though you will have already undergone an evaluation by your referring physician, the therapists who will be working with you will evaluate you as well to ensure they have a good perspective of your needs before designing your treatment plan. The evaluation is usually very extensive and can take about 90 minutes. During that time, you will be evaluated in a variety of areas, which may differ depending on the rehabilitation facility you attend. The evaluations may include (but not be limited to):

- Vital signs (heart rate and blood pressure).
- Range of motion.
- Posture.
- Strength in your extremities.
- Sensation testing in feet and ankles. While your eyes are closed, a therapist may use weighted calibrated filaments to touch your feet and ankles to determine the extent of sensation loss.
- Proprioception sensation. A therapist may test to see if your body can tell which position your joints are in, for example, when standing on an uneven surface such as sand or grass.
- Nystagmus testing (similar to electronystagmography; see chapter 2).
- Screen for BPPV using the Dix-Hallpike maneuver.

- Static balance (Romberg test).
- Balance testing (stand on foam and on one leg).
- Dynamic balance. A therapist may watch while you walk at different speeds, while looking up and down or while making turns.
- Gait. A therapist may watch to see whether you shuffle, stumble, or sway when you walk.

A therapist will also ask you about your lifestyle. Do you have a job that requires you to move your head from side to side? Do you need to climb stairs at home or at work? Do you do any lifting or reaching overhead? Do you walk on uneven city streets, grass, or other yielding surfaces that may present a balance problem? Do you drive (or did you drive and want to return to driving)? A goal of therapy is to help you return to as normal and functional a lifestyle as possible.

A therapist may also conduct an assessment of your living environment to make sure it is safe, and ask if there are any family members or other reliable individuals who can help you with your home exercise program, if needed. Overall, the evaluation lets your therapist know the areas in which you need assistance and the movements to which you are sensitive. Using all the information gathered, your therapist will devise your rehabilitation program.

How to Find a Vestibular Rehabilitation Therapy Facility

In most cases, physicians refer their patients to a vestibular rehabilitation facility with which they have a relationship. Hundreds of such centers are located across the United States, and you're likely to find several in most large cities. Often these facilities are part of a hospital, medical center, or medical school, but many are privately run. To locate physicians and physical therapists who are involved in vestibular rehabilitation therapy, as well as rehabilitation centers, you can contact VEDA at www.vestibular.org/resources.html where you can obtain contact information by state.

Exercises You Can Do at Home

Once your therapist has made an evaluation of your specific needs, he or she (along with other team members as needed) will design an exercise rehabilitation program for you that includes exercises you are to do at home daily. At the vestibular rehabilitation center, your therapist will teach and guide you through each of the exercises until you are comfortable doing them. You will be given written instructions, with illustrations of the exercises as needed. (Illustrations are especially helpful for people who may have some memory problems or who have trouble picturing verbal descriptions.) If you need any instruction on how to use certain devices, such as a cane or walker, you will be assisted with that as well. You may be asked to keep a daily diary of when you do your exercises and how you respond.

Below are some examples of the types of exercises you may be asked to do at home. Your therapist will tell you how many times you should do each exercise daily; twice is usually the minimum. You may need to have someone stay with you while you perform these exercises in case you lose your balance or need assistance.

Note: For your safety, we recommend that you consult with your physician and/or physical therapist before beginning any type of exercise program. A therapist can determine which level of exercise you can begin with and when you're ready to progress to the next level, the different types of exercises that will serve you best, and whether it is safe for you to do them by yourself.

HEAD MOVEMENT EXERCISES

These exercises help improve the vestibular-ocular reflex; in other words, the synchronization between your visual and vestibular systems.

1. While sitting in a sturdy chair, hold a card on which you've printed a single letter in your hand and extend your arm straight out in front of you so the card is at eye level. Look at the letter on the card, then bend your head forward, and then bend it backward, always keeping your eyes focused on the letter on the card. Begin slowly and try to keep the card or letter from appearing to shake or jiggle. If you are able to keep the card from appearing to move, repeat the exercise, this time increasing the speed at which you move your head.
2. Repeat the entire exercise, but this time move your head from side to side.
3. Repeat both (1) and (2), but this time stand on a firm surface and keep your feet shoulder width apart.
4. Gradually try to perform each exercise for up to 2 minutes.
5. Repeat both (1) and (2), but this time stand with your feet together.
6. Repeat both (1) and (2) while standing with your feet tandem (one foot directly in front of the other).
7. Repeat both (1) and (2) while standing on a compliant surface (e.g., a pillow or foam).

SITTING EXERCISES

- While sitting in a sturdy chair, shrug your shoulders 20 times.
- Turn your shoulders to the left, then to the right 20 times each side.
- Keeping your back straight, bend over and pick up objects from the ground in front of your chair (e.g., marbles, spools

of thread, or pencils) and sit up. If dizziness occurs, wait until it subsides, then repeat the exercise again 5 times.

GUIDED WALKING EXERCISES

- Choose a long hallway (at least 15 feet long) where you can walk while touching the wall. Touch the wall with your hand and maintain contact with it as you walk to the end of the hall. Turn around and go back while touching the other wall with your other hand.
- When you can walk up and back without stumbling or bumping into the wall or leaning against it for support, try walking up and down the hall with your arms at your sides, not touching the wall but staying close to it.
- When you are comfortable walking next to the wall, try walking down the middle of the hall without using your hands or the wall for balance.

WALKABOUT EXERCISES

- Walk outside at a comfortable pace, turning your head from side to side to observe the view. Focus on a stationary object in front of you to fight off dizziness. Begin with a short walk (5 to 10 minutes) and build up to a 30-minute one.
- Find a mild slope (e.g., a driveway) that is clear of obstacles and walk up and down the slope with your eyes open, then closed, 10 times. You should have a spotter with you.

STANDING EXERCISES

- Using a sturdy chair with arms, go from a sitting to a standing position and back again 20 times with your eyes open. Try not to use the arms of the chair to push yourself up; or, if you must use them, do so as little as possible. (This exercise is often prescribed by therapists for elderly people to help build strength in the lower extremities.) Repeat the exercise with your eyes closed.

The next standing exercise works your visual and proprioceptive systems together.

- While standing, toss a small rubber ball from hand to hand just above eye level.

EYE DIZZINESS EXERCISE

This exercise is helpful if you get dizzy when you move your eyes, even if you are holding your head completely still.

- Lie down with your eyes closed. Slowly rotate them around as far up, down, and to both sides as you can.
- If one position causes you to become dizzy, keep your eyes in that position for up to a count of 10.
- Open your eyes and focus on a target. When the dizziness subsides, close your eyes and turn them to the direction that made you dizzy.

POSTURE CONTROL EXERCISES

These exercises can help you improve your balance and posture. Do them while barefoot or while wearing flat shoes. The surface should be a bare floor or a lightweight carpet.

- Stand next to a counter or other support surface in tandem. While your eyes are open, place your right foot directly in front of your left foot, with your right heel touching your left toes. Stay in this position for 30 seconds. Then switch and place your left foot directly in front of your right foot, with your left heel touching your right toes. Remain immobile for 30 seconds. Repeat the entire exercise with your eyes closed.

- Walk in tandem. While your eyes are open, place your right foot directly in front of your left foot, with your right heel touching your left toes. Bring your left foot forward and place the left heel directly in front of and touching your right toes. Continue in this fashion for 15 to 20 feet. Repeat with your eyes closed (make sure there are no obstacles in your way).
- Stand next to a support surface for safety and swing. While your eyes are open, stand on your left foot and gently swing your right foot back and forth as far as you can without touching the foot to the floor. Count how many times you swing your right foot. Then switch feet and count again. Repeat the entire exercise with your eyes closed and count the swings again.

GAIT EXERCISE

This exercise helps improve gait and balance.

- Place two sturdy chairs about 10 feet apart. Begin at one chair and walk to the other.
- When you reach the second chair, sit down without using your hands. Wait 5 seconds and then get up without using your hands.
- Walk back to the first chair, place your hand on the top of it, and stand on one leg for 5 seconds.
- Begin the cycle again and repeat it 9 more times.
- Repeat the entire exercise, but this time look side to side while you're walking. Repeat 9 more times.

Dizziness and Daily Life: How to Cope

Dizziness and balance problems can put a real damper on your life if you let them. Claudette is a 43-year-old paralegal who has

Ménière's disease. For a while she didn't tell her family about her condition, and she would make excuses to them and her friends. "I'd say I wasn't feeling well or was too busy to join them for a hike or for a trip to the museum. Then they stopped asking me to join them, and I felt bad, so I told them the truth. I just said, 'I have Ménière's disease, I get very dizzy sometimes, and I can't always predict when it's going to happen.' And they understood. So now I go out more often and I'm more relaxed because they know and understand."

Emotional support from a partner and family, friends, and coworkers is important if you are living with dizziness or a balance problem. Vestibular rehabilitation therapy can also play a major role, because it provides physical as well as emotional assistance from a team of experts. They, along with your doctor, can help you take control of your life.

Control of her life was exactly what Lila wanted when she began vestibular rehabilitation therapy. At 80 years old, she was in relatively good health, but she was suffering with age-related deterioration of her vision and balance system. "I needed a tune up," she says. "The physical therapist taught me some strength exercises, and the occupational therapist went over a lot of hints to help me around the house. I feel a lot safer and confident now."

We've taken the liberty of listing some of the useful hints therapists may offer to help you learn to cope with the everyday things that can be disruptive when you're trying to maintain balance (see box).

TAKING CARE OF YOURSELF: WAYS TO PREVENT DIZZINESS AND FALLS

Learning ways to cope with dizziness and prevent falls is an integral part of vestibular rehabilitation therapy. Here are some guidelines for you to consider for yourself or your loved ones:

- Sign up with an emergency response service. Some communities offer low-cost service for older adults.
- Inspect all carpeting in your home to ensure it is securely attached to the floor and is without wrinkles or turned up edges.
- Remove throw rugs from living areas.
- Use a cane or walker if you have severe problems walking.
- Walk daily if possible. Walking is an excellent exercise to maintain balance and strength.
- Wear sturdy, flat shoes with crepe soles. Athletic and walking shoes are a good choice. Avoid heels and open-toed shoes if balance is a problem.
- Keep all electric and telephone cords taped down or tucked away from walking or sitting areas.
- Install safety grab bars in the bathtub and shower walls. Ordinary towel bars and soap dishes are not strong enough to prevent a fall.
- Put nonskid strips in the bottom of the bathtub and shower stall.
- Use a shower chair in the shower or a bath bench in the bathtub.
- Use long-handled brooms, mops, and vacuum cleaner attachments that allow you not to have to bend over or twist your head.
- Sit while you brush your teeth, put on makeup, or shave.
- Keep all rooms and stairways well lit and clear of obstacles.
- Use nightlights. Also keep a light at your bedside so you can turn it on before getting out of bed in the middle of the night.
- Place brightly colored tape on the edge of the top and bottom steps of all stairs in and outside your home.

- If you wear eyeglasses or contacts, keep your prescription current. A poor prescription can contribute to your balance and dizziness problems.
- Always use the handrails when walking up or down stairs. If you come to stairs that have no rail, place your hand on the wall as you use the stairs or avoid using them at all.
- When you get up from a lying position, sit up slowly, wait a minute or two until you feel stable, then stand up slowly and stand still for a few seconds before you try to walk.
- When you need to change position, do so slowly and have something sturdy to hold onto in case you begin to feel dizzy or to lose your balance.
- In the kitchen or other rooms that have cabinets or shelves, place frequently used items on shelves that are easiest to reach. If you need to reach up or bend down to retrieve items, use a long-handled pole with an attachment that allows you to grab objects. Such tools can be found in catalogues that offer adaptive equipment (see appendix C), or ask your physical therapist or physician.
- Keep a cordless telephone next to your bed. Besides eliminating the need to go to another room to answer the phone, you can use it to make an emergency call should you fall when getting out of bed.
- If you need help getting out of chairs, consider chairs that have arm rests.

Maneuvers for Treatment of BPPV

Benign paroxysmal positional vertigo is one of the most common causes of vertigo and dizziness: about 25 percent of people who have a vestibular disorder suffer with BPPV. The good news is, it is also a condition that responds exceptionally well to one of three different, five-minute treatments that your physician or vestibular therapist can perform at your bedside or in the office. They are the Epley maneuver (named after its originator, J. M. Epley, M.D.; also known as the canalith repositioning treatment), the Semont (liberatory) maneuver, and the Brandt-Daroff treatment.

Although most people who have BPPV recover eventually without treatment, it isn't possible to know whether the wait will be weeks or months. Therefore, these noninvasive treatments can dramatically and immediately (in the case of the Epley and Semont maneuvers) improve the lives of people who are experiencing this type of inner ear problem. If BPPV should recur, which it sometimes does months or even years after the first episode, treatment with one of these maneuvers can be repeated.

The purpose of these maneuvers is to dislodge the free-floating debris (ear rocks) in one of the semicircular canals, which cause vertigo, and move them into an area where they won't cause vertigo.

EPLEY MANEUVER

This maneuver is used on patients who have severe vertigo. In 80 percent of patients, only one treatment is needed to eliminate symptoms. The maneuver has five steps (see figure 2, page 206), and you will remain in each position for about 60 seconds.

Some doctors place a vibrating device on the back of the ear (this is painless) to help move the debris.

SEMONT MANEUVER

The Semont maneuver involves very rapid movements from side to side; this makes it a less desirable choice for elderly individuals. Its success rate after one treatment has been reported to be 53 percent, and 76 to 90 percent after two treatments, usually done several weeks apart. The procedure is done in four steps:

1. You sit on the edge of a bed or treatment table.

Figure 2. Epley Maneuver

1. and 2. While you are sitting on a bed or examining table, the doctor will move you to a reclining position. Your head will be placed over the end of the bed or table at a 45-degree angle.

3. The doctor will turn your head to the opposite side.

4. You will be rolled over onto that side. Your head will be angled slightly so that you will be looking at the floor.

5. You will be returned to a sitting position. Your chin will be tilted down.

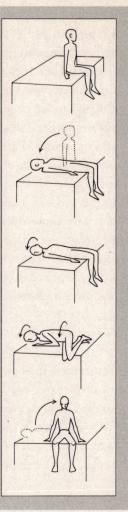

2. The doctor moves you quickly from the seated position to lie on the affected side. You stay in this position for three minutes.

3. The doctor then quickly moves you to lie on the opposite side. You stay in this position for three minutes.

4. You are slowly moved to a seated position.

BRANDT-DAROFF TREATMENT

Unlike the Epley and Semont maneuvers, the Brandt-Daroff treatment is done at home by the patient and repeated twice a day for one to two weeks. It is usually reserved for people who have mild residual symptoms after undergoing the Epley maneuver or who cannot tolerate that maneuver.

This treatment involves the following steps:

1. Sit on the side of the bed, then from the seated position, lie down on the side that causes the vertigo.
2. Maintain that position until the vertigo subsides.
3. Sit up and lie down on the opposite side; maintain this position for one to two minutes or until the vertigo subsides.
4. Repeat 1 through 3 five times in the morning when you get up and five times at night.

AFTER-TREATMENT CARE

After your doctor or therapist has done either the Epley or the Semont maneuver, wait ten minutes after the maneuver is completed before leaving the office to allow the ear rocks to reposition themselves. Do not drive; arrange to have someone pick you up. For at least two days, follow these precautions:

• Sleep with your head at a 45-degree angle. You can either sleep in a recliner or a bed that can be positioned at this angle. Sleeping with a lot of pillows to prop you up often does not work because many people toss and turn during the night and end up in a flat or near-flat position.
• During the day, keep your head vertical.
• Do not go to the hairdresser or dentist, because their chairs recline and cause your head to lean back.
• Avoid any exercises that require you to move your head. Riding a stationary bike, for example, would be safe; playing tennis would not.

- If you need to use eyedrops, do so without tilting your head back.

For the next five days after the first two posttreatment days, follow these procedures:

- Avoid sleeping on the side with the affected ear.
- Use two pillows under your head when you sleep.
- Stay as upright as possible. If you must go to the dentist, ask if the chair can remain upright.
- Avoid exercises that extend the neck or head, such as sit-ups or touching your toes.

One week after your treatment, carefully move into the position that usually makes you dizzy. Have a friend stand by in case you start to fall. Return to your doctor for a follow-up evaluation. If the treatment was not successful, you will need a repeat maneuver.

Tai Chi

Tai chi is an ancient Chinese technique that combines healing, and meditation in a slow-moving, gentle series of movements. In the United States, it is popular as a way to improve balance, relieve tension and anxiety, and achieve inner calm and harmony.

Traditional tai chi consists of more than 100 movements, but the modern, abbreviated form includes 24 to 48. Every move is gentle and natural and performed the way the body was designed to move. Therefore there is no strain or unnatural pressure placed on the body. This makes tai chi an excellent exercise for people of all ages and abilities. In fact, more than a dozen studies show that tai chi is especially helpful for older adults who want to improve balance and help prevent falls.

One ten-year study conducted by Emory, Harvard, and Yale

Universities found that tai chi reduced the risk of injury from falling by 48 percent. A study funded by the National Institutes of Health and sponsored by Northwestern University in Chicago found that tai chi significantly improved balance among people who had mild balance disorders.

Both the National Institutes of Health and the National Institute on Aging recognize tai chi as a way to significantly reduce the risk of falls among older individuals. It can be an excellent complementary therapy to use along with a vestibular rehabilitation program. Talk to your physician and physical therapist about including tai chi as part of your therapy. Your tai chi instructor should be informed of any balance problems you are experiencing. If possible, find a tai chi group that focuses on individuals who have balance problems.

Bottom Line

Vestibular therapies can help the body heal itself. The Epley and related maneuvers for BPPV are testimony to the amazing ability of the body to regain harmony, with the aid of some very simple yet effective moves. Another example of the power of simplicity is tai chi, which can be beneficial to nearly anyone who wants to improve or maintain their balance.

Vestibular rehabilitation therapy can speed up recovery from vestibular damage, increase strength and range of motion, improve balance, and get you back on the road to independence in a matter of weeks. It can be especially helpful for elderly individuals who often must learn to cope with declining visual, proprioceptive, and vestibular function. A referral from a physician who is familiar with your specific needs and medical condition can get you into a program near you.

13

Treating Dizziness with Diet

What you eat has a significant impact on every function in your body, and the inner ear is no exception. Even though the inner ear contains only a minute amount of fluid, we've already seen how critically important it is to maintain inner ear health, especially when it comes to dizziness, vertigo, and disequilibrium. Certain nutritional factors play a role in that goal. In this chapter we talk about some simple dietary changes you can make, beginning right now, that may have a positive impact on your dizziness and balance problems.

Every year, millions of Americans visit their doctors in search of help for problems relating to dizziness, vertigo, and/or disequilibrium. That probably doesn't surprise you, because you're probably one of those millions. And if you're like most of those individuals, you're hoping your doctor will hand you a "magic bullet" at the end of your visit.

In many cases, however, simple dietary changes can provide most or all of the relief you need from dizziness. That's not to say that appropriate medications don't have their place. In fact, diuretics are often prescribed along with dietary changes, as we discuss in this chapter. But isn't it good to know that there are some easy dietary changes you can make right now that may relieve your lightheadedness and dizziness? You'll learn all about them in the pages ahead.

Monitor Salt Intake

A healthy tip for *anyone* who experiences vertigo is to reduce the amount of sodium in his or her diet. This advice is especially important for people who have Ménière's disease. In fact, a combination of a low-salt diet and short-term use of diuretics is the only treatment many people with Ménière's disease need to get relief. It is the first recommendation I give to my patients who have this inner ear disorder. This combination approach can also be beneficial for people who have perilymphatic fistula or vestibular neuronitis with recurrent symptoms.

Sodium and Salt

Most people believe sodium and salt are one and the same, but they are not. Salt is a compound that contains 40 percent sodium and 60 percent chloride. When you look at an ingredient label to see how much salt is in a specific food, you'll see "sodium" and not "salt" on the list. Keep this in mind when you begin to check your food products for their salt content. It is the amount of sodium in your diet that you want to reduce.

One-half teaspoon of salt contains approximately 1,100 milligrams (mg) of sodium. Although this doesn't sound like much, it's more than your body needs to function properly: 500 milligrams daily is the minimum requirement. Yet most Americans consume 2,500 to 5,000 milligrams of sodium per day, up to more than four times the daily recommended amount. To help eliminate dizziness, you'll need to keep your daily intake to 2,000 milligrams or less, and we're going to show you how.

REDUCING YOUR SODIUM INTAKE

Our taste for salt is acquired. That means, now that your taste buds have learned to taste salt, they can learn to adjust to less salt. You can gradually reduce your use of salt so the change won't make your adjustment too difficult. However, you will likely notice better results with dizziness if you make a more aggressive reduction in your salt intake.

To successfully—and less painfully—reduce your salt intake, you need to follow a few simple guidelines.

- Read the "Nutritional Information" labels on all your foods. You may be surprised at the amount of sodium in the foods you eat. Canned and packaged dinners are especially high in sodium. Make sure you calculate the milligrams for the number of servings you eat. If one serving of canned corn contains 310 milligrams of sodium, and the whole can contains three servings, then the entire can has 930 milligrams of sodium. If you eat two servings, you've consumed 620 milligrams.
- Look for foods labeled "salt-free" or "sodium-free." Those marked "low sodium" or "reduced sodium" may contain more sodium than you think. (See "What Does 'Low Salt' or 'Low Sodium' Really Mean?" below.)
- Do not put a salt shaker on the table. Replace it with a pepper shaker or spices and herbs to flavor your food.
- Make liberal use of strong, nonsodium flavorings, such as lemon or lime juice, vinegar, freshly grated horseradish, minced fresh garlic, and chopped onions to help you kick the salt habit.
- Avoid processed foods as much as possible. Instead, cook from scratch, using natural, fresh ingredients that are natu-

rally low in sodium, like fresh fruits and vegetables, whole grains, beans, and legumes.

- When making recipes from scratch, identify those which include salt as an ingredient. In most cases, you can completely eliminate the salt or use a substitute. For example, when making pie crust, you can use ¼ teaspoon cider vinegar instead of ¼ teaspoon salt. To find other low- or no-salt recipes, see Suggested Readings.
- Drink lots of water, but when choosing bottled water, make sure you select sodium-free or low-sodium varieties. Some bottled waters contain up to 250 milligrams of sodium per 8 ounces.
- Choose seltzer water instead of club soda. Club soda contains sodium chloride and sodium bicarbonate (baking soda), two types of sodium you don't need.
- Avoid adding salt to cooking water when you're making pasta, beans, and grains. Instead, add some fresh herbs, a bay leaf, or some fresh lemon juice to the water. When making cooked cereals, add caraway or anise seeds or a bit of minced fresh ginger instead of salt.
- Eat fresh or frozen (no salt added) vegetables instead of canned or jarred.
- Avoid salty foods such as pickles, salty snacks, salted nuts, processed meats and fish (luncheon meats, sausage, pepperoni, and canned fish such as sardines and tuna), and canned soups (except for low-salt varieties).
- Watch your condiments. Ketchup, mustard, steak sauce, and soy sauce all contain high amounts of salt.
- Avoid the flavor enhancer monosodium glutamate (MSG). It contains 12 percent sodium.
- If you use wine when cooking, use table or drinking wine or sherry. Cooking wine and cooking sherry have added salt.
- Make your own air-popped, unsalted popcorn, and season it with garlic or onion powder (not garlic or onion salt) or your

favorite herbs, or sprinkle it with nutritional yeast, which will give it a buttery flavor.

- If you love nuts, you can still enjoy them by getting unsalted, dry roasted varieties and sprinkling them with garlic or onion powder.
- When you eat out, insist that your food be made without added salt. Ask for lemon, garlic powder, onion powder, oregano and other herbs, or pepper on the side, or bring these seasonings with you from home in a shaker.
- Consider using a salt substitute (e.g., Mrs. Dash, Lipton, Precision Foods). Because these substitutes are high in potassium, you should check with your doctor before using them if you have kidney problems, are taking medications to treat heart failure or high blood pressure, or have other medical conditions.
- If you take over-the-counter medications, check the label for their sodium content. If you take prescription medications, ask the pharmacist for that information.

WHAT DOES "LOW SALT" OR "LOW SODIUM" REALLY MEAN?

You've probably seen many labels and packages that proclaim the food is "no salt" or "low salt," or "low sodium," or "reduced sodium." What do these phrases really mean? You may be surprised.

- Sodium- or salt-free: less than 5 milligrams of sodium per serving.
- Very low sodium: 35 milligrams or less per serving.
- Low sodium: 140 milligrams or less per serving.
- Reduced sodium: at least 25 percent less sodium than the regular variety.
- Unsalted or no salt added: no salt has been added to the food item during processing, but this does not mean the product

is sodium-free. The "unsalted" or "no salt added" label can be especially misleading, so be sure to read the nutritional panel information.

HOW SALTY IS THAT?

Some foods can provide you with nearly an entire day's allowance of salt in one serving. Fast foods are notorious for this. Here are just a few common foods and their sodium content. Remember to always read the nutritional information on the foods you buy. The sodium content of fast foods can usually be found on each individual company's website under "Nutritional Information."

FOOD ITEM	Sodium (mg)
Apple, raw	1
Bacon (Canadian) 3.5 oz	2,500
Bouillon cube (1)	1,200
Carrot, 1/4 cup cooked	25
Celery, 1 stalk	70
Cheese, 1 oz	200–500
Crackers, saltines 3.5 oz	1,100
Ham, 1 oz	300–500
Ketchup, 1 tb	150–200
McDonald's hamburger	590
McDonald's Big Mac	1,090
McDonald's large fries	350
McDonald's McNuggets, 9 pieces	1,020
McDonald's ham, egg & cheese bagel	1,490
Mustard, 1 tsp	65–80
Olive, 1 medium	35–100

Orange juice, 3.5 oz	1
Peaches	2
Peanut butter, 2 tb	150–200
Pizza Hut, 1 slice pepperoni	390
Pizza Hut, stuffed crust, cheese	1,090
Pizza Hut, stuffed crust, sausage	1,180
Pizza Hut, personal pan, 1 cheese	1,370
Pizza Hut, personal pan, 1 sausage	1,640
Spinach, 1/2 cup	30–65
Tuna, 1/3 cup	250–325

Cut the Caffeine

That first cup of coffee in the morning may give you a lift but it also constricts your blood vessels, and this can impair the circulation to your inner ear. The result can be unsteadiness or light-headedness. Reducing or eliminating caffeine from your diet may greatly improve your dizziness.

Some people switch to decaffeinated coffee (and tea or cola) because they like the taste of these beverages but want to avoid the caffeine. The decaffeination process does not remove 100 percent of the caffeine, but the remaining amount is reported to be around 2 percent, which is negligible.

Breaking free of a caffeine habit (caffeine is habit-forming but not addictive) can be a challenge if you're among those who drink several cups of coffee (or caffeinated tea or cola) daily. Withdrawal symptoms can include severe headache, restlessness, depression, poor concentration, lethargy, irritability, and flu-like symptoms within 18 to 24 hours of stopping.

The best way to kick the habit is to do so gradually: reduce your intake of caffeine by about 20 percent per week over a four-to-five-week period. For example, if you drink five cups of coffee or five cans of cola daily, reduce your intake to four cups (or cans) the first week, three the second week, and so on. To get an idea of how much caffeine you are ingesting, see the box.

CAFFEINE LEVELS OF BEVERAGES

Coffee (brewed)	110–150 mg per 5 oz
Coffee (instant)	40–108 mg per 5 oz
Black tea	20–50 mg per 5 oz
Green tea	20–50 mg per 5 oz
Iced tea	22–36 mg per 12 oz
Hot cocoa	2–8 mg per 6 oz
Chocolate bar	11 mg per 1.55 oz
Coca-Cola	46 mg per 12 oz
Pepsi-Cola	38 mg per 12 oz
Jolt soft drink	72 mg per 12 oz

More than 1,000 over-the-counter (OTC) drugs contain caffeine, ranging from "stay-awake" pills (which are often pure caffeine) to pain relievers to cold remedies to weight control products. Check labels of all OTC drugs before you take them if you are concerned about caffeine. Here's the caffeine content of just a few OTC drugs: All amounts are per tablet:

NoDoz	100 mg
Vivarin	200 mg
Anacin	32 mg
Excedrin	65 mg
Excedrin PM	0 mg
Midol	32 mg
Vanquish	33 mg

Other Dietary Tips

These dietary tips have proved beneficial for many people. Incorporate one or more of them into your routine to see if they are helpful to you.

• Reduce sugar intake. Consumption of simple sugars—table sugar, brown sugar, honey, corn syrup, molasses, candy—cause your blood sugar levels to rise quickly, and then fall. Some experts believe that wide fluctuations in blood sugar levels have an adverse effect on the fluids in the inner ear. In people who are susceptible to dizziness or who have an inner ear problem, these fluctuations may cause dizziness. Experiment with this idea: Make notes in your diary about your sugar consumption and see if you notice any difference in lightheadedness or dizziness based on your sugar consumption.

• Avoid monosodium glutamate (MSG). This taste enhancer is probably best known for its use in Chinese restaurant foods, yet many have now stopped using it. People who are intolerant of MSG may experience headache, nausea, vomiting, balance problems, asthma attacks, anxiety or panic attacks, runny nose, mouth lesions, and depression. Read labels carefully. Even if the label doesn't list MSG specifically, other ingredients contain MSG, including hydrolyzed protein, autolyzed yeast, yeast extract, sodium or calcium caseinate, and gelatin. Others that may contain MSG (depending on the manufacturer) include textured protein, vegetable gum, carrageenan, whey protein, whey protein isolate, and barley malt.

• Help maintain bodily fluids at a constant level by drinking water regularly throughout the day. Keep several water bottles filled and refrigerated at all times. If you are using purchased bottled water, make sure it is sodium-free.

• Check to see if you have food allergies. Some people get dizzy for no apparent reason, and then discover that they are reacting to specific foods. You can uncover food allergies by maintaining a food diary as part of your journal for a week or so: keep a record of all the foods and beverages you consume and note any dizzy episodes. If you see a link between a certain food and dizziness, eliminate that food for several weeks to see if the dizzy spells return. You may be allergic to more than one food. Foods that are most likely to cause allergic reactions are milk, wheat, peanuts, tomatoes, oranges, mushrooms, and fish. You can also ask your doctor to conduct allergy testing to determine which foods may be causing you a problem. There are several tests doctors can perform to identify food allergies and sensitivities. Discuss this possibility with your health-care provider.

•   If you experience migraines, foods that may trigger attacks include alcohol, aged cheeses, avocado, bananas, caffeine, chicken liver, chocolate, citrus, dairy foods, nuts, onions, pickled herring, sour cream, yeast and yeast extracts, yogurt, and food additives such as monosodium glutamate, aspartame (artificial sweetener), and nitrates (found in luncheon meats and hot dogs). Avoid these foods.

Bottom Line

When the situation is appropriate, I believe in beginning with the simplest therapies first, and dietary change is the place to start for anyone who is experiencing dizziness. The suggestions offered in this chapter can benefit anyone; the worst they can do is provide no relief. If you have Ménière's disease, or if you're experiencing dizziness, vertigo, and/or migraine you suspect may be associated with food allergies or sensitivities, try the recommendations we've proposed, keep a record in your diary of the foods you eliminate and add, and note any reactions you have. You may be able to eat your dizziness away.

14

Surgical and Medical Procedures

If you've turned to this chapter, chances are your doctor has already mentioned that you may or should consider surgery for your condition. The majority of people who have vertigo or a vestibular disorder eventually recover given time, patience, dietary changes, medication, and/or vestibular rehabilitation therapy. However, a small percentage of people who have a vestibular condition that has not responded to other treatment approaches elects surgery. Thus surgery is generally reserved for people who have severely debilitating cases of Ménière's disease, vestibular neuritis, and in some cases, otosclerosis or benign paroxysmal positional vertigo. In this chapter we explain the various surgical options for these conditions.

You can use the information in this chapter to help prepare you for your discussion with your doctor. As you read this chapter, you will probably think of some questions you'll want to ask your doctor, so keep a list of them to take with you to the office.

Types of Surgical and Medical Procedures

Surgical procedures for dizziness and balance disorders fall into two general categories: conservative (nondestructive) and destructive. Whenever possible, surgeons choose to do nondestructive procedures. These are done in an attempt to preserve a person's hearing and remaining vestibular function, although there is still a chance that hearing will be lost. In some people, for example, hearing continues to deteriorate after they've had a surgical procedure to eliminate vertigo. The progression of hearing loss is based on the natural history of the disease. This is a possibility you need to discuss with your doctor.

If you have debilitating or severe vertigo and poor or severely damaged hearing, your doctor may recommend a procedure in which he or she deliberately destroys your balance system and/or your hearing. This may sound like a drastic measure to take, but in some cases it is necessary for people to lose their hearing to eliminate debilitating vertigo. Fortunately, the brain has the ability to compensate, and the balance function returns. We discuss several destructive surgical procedures below.

DESTRUCTIVE PROCEDURES

Chemical Labyrinthectomy. This procedure is used by some physicians to treat Ménière's disease. A chemical labyrinthectomy can be done in a doctor's office and requires only a local anesthetic applied to the eardrum. There are different ways to apply the treatment to the inner ear. A needle could be used to introduce the antibiotic gentamicin into the middle ear. The patient is then asked to lie on the opposite ear for 20 to 25 minutes to allow the gentamicin to be absorbed into the inner ear. There are different protocols for the frequency of these injections. The number of treatments is determined according to response of symptoms and side effects. Side effects include temporary imbalance and mild hearing loss. Vestibular rehabilitation exercises can help minimize any balance problems that you encounter after the procedure.

Another type of chemical labyrinthectomy for Ménière's disease involves delivering the gentamicin to the inner ear via a small wick or a catheter. Whichever way gentamicin is delivered to the inner ear, the effect is the same. Gentamicin typically destroys the balance cells in the inner ear, but it will also destroy the hearing cells at higher doses.

The majority of people adjust to the complete loss of balance nerve function with the aid of vestibular rehabilitation therapy, which helps the brain compensate for the loss. An advantage of chemical labyrinthectomy using gentamicin injection is that many people don't experience any additional hearing loss.

Labyrinthectomy. "When my doctor told me nearly 100 percent of people who undergo a labyrinthectomy are free of vertigo attacks, I said that was the operation for me." Roxanne, a 49-year-old mother of three had been living with Ménière's disease for about two years when she sat down with her doctor to discuss surgery. She had already given up her executive position with a Fortune 500 company because she could no longer function at work. Now she was confined to the house most of the time, and she was depressed, anxious, and desperate for relief.

Roxanne was a good candidate for labyrinthectomy. The disease was confined to her left ear, and she had lost about 80 percent of hearing in that ear. Her right ear was unaffected. This was important, because labyrinthectomy destroys the labyrinth; this means the ear that undergoes the operation loses all hearing and balance function. While the brain can compensate for the loss of balance, with the help of vestibular rehabilitation therapy, the hearing is gone forever.

I explained to Roxanne that during the procedure, I would remove the semicircular canals and the vestibule in her left ear. This would leave her completely deaf in that ear, but vertigo would likely be eliminated. The procedure would take about one hour and would be done under general anesthesia.

Roxanne underwent the procedure, and after surgery she experienced some vertigo for a day or two, which we controlled with meclizine. Such episodes of vertigo are normal after this procedure, until the brain is able to compensate for the loss of vestibular information from the operated ear. During the next eight weeks, Roxanne participated in vestibular rehabilitation therapy, which accelerated her recovery by helping her brain learn to compensate for the loss of vestibular function in her left ear. Roxanne went back to work one month after surgery.

A variation of the surgical approach I discussed with Roxanne is to drill a channel in the bone between the round and oval windows. This destroys the inner ear and also results in hearing loss. It is not as predictable in eliminating vertigo, however, because some inner ear balance cells are left behind. This partial labyrinthectomy is sometimes used for elderly patients because the procedure takes less time and requires less recovery time.

Vestibular Neurectomy (Vestibular Nerve Section). If you have debilitating vertigo from Ménière's disease but your hearing has not been affected, a vestibular neurectomy may be your surgical answer. This procedure involves cutting the vestibular nerve, which runs between the ear and the brain, in the section that controls balance while preserving the section that controls hearing. So while this procedure completely eliminates vestibular function in the operated ear, hearing is preserved. Ninety to ninety-five percent of people who undergo this procedure, which takes about three hours, are cured of vertigo.

Recovery time is about four to six weeks and could include vestibular rehabilitation therapy to help the brain compensate for the loss of the vestibular nerve function. Vestibular neurectomy is usually best for individuals who have disabling vertigo and good residual hearing in the affected ear and who are younger than 70 years old and in good health.

NONDESTRUCTIVE PROCEDURES

Endolymphatic Sac Surgery. The first endolymphatic sac surgical procedure on humans was performed in 1927, and today it is probably the most common operation done for people who need surgery for Ménière's disease. The procedure is based on the principle that there is too much endolymphatic fluid in the inner ear, and this excess fluid causes the compartment of the inner ear to swell and vertigo to occur

If you decide to undergo endolymphatic sac surgery, your doctor will place a drain, or *shunt*, in your ear, which will allow the excess fluid to continuously leave the inner ear and thus reduce the swelling and eliminate the vertigo. Surgery successfully controls vertigo in up to 70 percent of the patients if they have the procedure done early in the course of the disease. The success rate drops to about 55 percent if they've had symptoms of Ménière's disease for five years. The incidence of hearing loss as a side effect of surgery is about 1 to 7 percent.

Cochleosacculotomy. The aim of this surgical procedure is to relieve pressure in the inner ear of people who have Ménière's disease. Because cochleosacculotomy can be done under local anesthesia, it was a popular procedure among elderly patients who are at high risk if placed under general anesthesia. The procedure takes about one hour.

During a cochleosacculotomy, the surgeon uses a small, sharp instrument to pierce the round window in the middle ear to reach the utricle. This allows the fluid to drain out and pressure to be relieved. Success rates (complete or nearly complete elimination of vertigo) of 88 percent have been reported, although there is a significant risk (65 percent) of mild to moderate hearing loss. Because of the great possibility of hearing loss, this procedure is often reserved for elderly patients who already have some hearing loss but for whom vertigo is a major concern, especially with the risk of falling and suffering a fracture. This procedure is not frequently performed anymore since similar results can be obtained with gentamicin injections.

Posterior Semicircular Canal Occlusion. Most people who have benign paroxysmal positional vertigo find that the condition resolves itself without treatment, usually within one year or they respond to a simple maneuver (Epley maneuver; see chapter 12) their doctor does in the office. But a small percentage of people with BPPV don't get better with either of these possibilities, and their debilitating vertigo attacks persist. For them, a surgical procedure called posterior semicircular canal occlusion can help.

Harold, a 38-year-old general construction contractor, can attest to that. While trimming a tree in his backyard one day, he slipped and fell 6 feet to the ground, injuring his head. The injury caused BPPV, and despite several attempts with the Epley maneuver, his violent vertigo episodes continued and he was completely unable to work. I explained the procedure to Harold, and he agreed to have it. I made an incision behind the ear, located the posterior semicircular canal (which is the canal involved in BPPV), and plugged the canal with a special waxy material. This plug made the canal nonfunctional, and also eliminated Harold's vertigo attacks. He returned to work within a few days of surgery and has not experienced another vertigo episode.

Some people experience a little dizziness for a day or two after undergoing a posterior semicircular canal occlusion, but most suffer no side effects at all. Vestibular rehabilitation therapy is not needed for the majority of people, although elderly patients can benefit from a few sessions postsurgically.

Bottom Line

When vertigo doesn't respond to other treatment methods and it is having a devastating effect on your life, surgical options are available. If you and your doctor decide surgery is the best choice for you, be sure you thoroughly understand all the risks and benefits, what to expect during your recovery, and the side effects of the procedure before you have the surgery. Discuss and prepare a plan for how you will handle your recovery process, which will include vestibular rehabilitation therapy (discussed in chapter 12) and perhaps some complementary therapies as well, which we turn to in the next chapter.

15

Complementary Treatment Methods

Complementary treatments, such as herbal and homeopathic remedies and relaxation techniques, are yet more options you can explore in the treatment of your dizziness or balance problems. Regardless of the type of vestibular disorder you have, there's likely a complementary therapy that can help you. In this chapter, we introduce you to some complementary treatment approaches for dizziness, vertigo, and disequilibrium that can be used safely and effectively along with the more conventional approaches we've discussed in previous chapters.

Are Complementary Therapies for You?

How do you know if complementary therapies are for you? Some of the alternative treatments discussed in this chapter are for specific types of dizziness or balance problems, while others are more general in scope. For example, if your dizziness, vertigo, or disequilibrium is associated with an injury to the cervical spine (neck) area, then acupuncture or chiropractic may help you.

If your symptoms are associated with a psychological disorder, stress reduction and biofeedback approaches may be most helpful for you. However, these therapies can be helpful for anyone who is experiencing problems with dizziness, because stress can exacerbate your symptoms. In addition, herbal and homeopathic remedies are often beneficial if you are experiencing motion sickness, stress, or symptoms associated with dizziness and vertigo, such as nausea and vomiting.

Using Complementary Therapies

We remind you that the complementary treatments discussed in this chapter are just that: complementary. They are not meant to replace the medical advice of your health-care providers or any medication, surgical procedures, or vestibular rehabilitation exercises prescribed by them. Complementary methods can be powerful treatments and occasionally may not interact well with the medical treatments you are using. We have included precautions with the various complementary treatments discussed in this chapter; however, these warnings are not all-inclusive. Therefore it is critical that you talk to your doctors and therapists before starting any complementary treatment.

Acupuncture

Controversy exists as to whether acupuncture is effective in treating or preventing dizziness and vertigo. Although there are many positive anecdotal reports of its effectiveness, there are few scientific studies that support those claims. Among this latter group are several recent preliminary studies on the use of acupuncture for vertigo in more than 400 patients, in which it was successful in 95 percent of cases. In these individuals, the vertigo was associated with compression in the cervical spine. The effectiveness of acupuncture in other types of dizziness or vertigo has not been verified.

Acupuncture is an ancient Chinese medical system that is used to diagnose and treat a wide variety of physical and emotional ailments, as well as prevent disease and improve overall well-being. It has withstood the test of time: since it was first practiced more than 3,000 years ago, it has grown in popularity around the world.

The basis of acupuncture is its ability to stimulate the activity of the autonomic nervous system, which is responsible for the function of the internal organs, including the ear, as well as emotional states, such as depression, phobia, and anxiety. To achieve these effects, practitioners of acupuncture insert ultrathin needles into specific spots on the body in order to release blocked energy at those points. The energy is *chi*, which, according to traditional Chinese medicine, is the life force that flows through the body along invisible pathways called *meridians*. When practitioners release the energy at specific points, chi can flow freely and help return balance to the body and allow the body to heal itself. (To locate an acupuncture practitioner near you see appendix C.)

Biofeedback

Biofeedback is a method that allows you to use special devices, learned techniques, or both to get information about what is happening in your body, and then use that information to control or regulate certain internal functions. Thus, you can learn to control your response to stress by changing your heart rate, breathing rate, blood pressure, body temperature, and muscle contractions that may be causing you dizziness, anxiety, pain, or discomfort.

Although there are several types of biofeedback, the type most relevant to dizziness and balance disorders is thermal biofeedback. For this type, sensors are placed on the fingers to record skin temperature, which is an indication of amount of blood flow. The sensors send the information to a device, usually with a screen, that tells you what your skin temperature is. Your "job" is to use visualization or imagery techniques to bring the temperature up if it is too low; that is, imagine that your blood is flowing to your hands or feet. The "feedback" is in the form of flashing lights, beeps, or lines on a computer screen monitoring your body temperature. With practice and over several sessions, you should be able to increase the blood flow to your hands or feet. This type of biofeedback has proven useful for people who have poor circulation, migraine, anxiety, and temporomandibular disorder, all conditions that can play a role in dizziness, vertigo, and disequilibrium.

Another type of biofeedback is electromyographic biofeedback, in which sensors are placed over tense or painful muscles. Electromyographic biofeedback can help reduce anxiety. This time the feedback is about muscle tension, and you learn to mentally relax the muscles related to your anxiety and dizziness.

Biofeedback is best learned from a professional, who usually can be found at biofeedback or complementary medicine facilities. After you master the technique, you will be able to achieve the desired results without use of the recording device. For information about where to find biofeedback experts, ask your doctor or see appendix C.

Chiropractic

The joints in the neck (cervical area) play a role in the coordination of the head, eyes, and body, as well as in posture, equilibrium, and spatial orientation. When those joints become irritated or injured, due to whiplash, a fall, or other trauma that causes misalignment of the vertebrae in the neck and interference with the normal transmission of signals between the spinal cord and brain, dizziness, vertigo, ringing in the ears, disequilibrium, and nausea can result. Sometimes these symptoms occur immediately after the injury; other times days, weeks, or months may pass before they manifest. The diagnosis may include cervical vertigo, positional vertigo, or whiplash injuries.

TESTS CHIROPRACTORS MAY DO

Chiropractors can conduct several simple tests to determine whether your symptoms are caused by cervical trauma.

One test to determine whether disequilibrium is caused by a cervical problem is the Hautant's test. This test demonstrates the ability of the cervical spine to regulate muscle tone correctly in the legs and arms. The chiropractor will ask you to sit in a chair, preferably one that has good back support, and to hold your arms straight out in front of you, palms down. You will then close your eyes and remain in that position while the doctor watches to see if your arms drift to one side. You will then repeat the exercise, but this time you will turn your head to the left, and then to the right. In many cases, the amount of arm drift will be more obvious when the head is turned in the direction that matches the cervical injury.

Another test can be used to help identify cervical vertigo. You will be asked to sit on a rotating stool with your feet flat on the floor. The chiropractor will hold your head still while you twist side to side on the chair. By holding your head, the chiropractor prevents stimulation of the inner ear while allowing movement of the cervical spine. If vertigo occurs, he or she will suspect that your vertigo is associated with injury to your cervical spine.

CHIROPRACTIC TREATMENT

The type of chiropractic treatment that has proved helpful in relieving and eliminating the symptoms related to cervical spinal injury is called upper cervical (upper neck) chiropractic, an approach that incorporates computerized technology. Treatment typically consists of an examination of the spine, x-rays of the upper neck, computerized thermal spinal scans (which measure the amount of irritation to the nerves), and physical adjustments of the cervical spine to realign the vertebrae in the upper neck. The number and frequency of treatments will depend on the severity of your condition and your response.

Herbal and Nutritional Supplements

More and more, health-care providers and the general public are turning to herbal remedies as complementary or sole treatments for various ailments. Of the hundreds of herbs and nutrients at our disposal, there are several that may provide some relief from dizziness and vertigo and from the nausea, vomiting, and anxiety that often accompany them. Here are a few that have proven to be helpful for some people.

GINKGO BILOBA

Ginkgo biloba is an herb that comes from the leaves of the world's oldest surviving tree. This herb was used for millennia to treat asthma and digestive problems and to prevent drunkenness, but in recent decades scientists discovered that it is also effective in improving blood flow to the brain. This finding then led to studies in which investigators found that ginkgo can help improve memory and mental clarity, as well as be beneficial in the treatment of dizziness, ringing in the ears, and anxiety.

Ginkgo should not be used if you are taking any other substance that thins the blood, such as aspirin, warfarin (Coumadin), or clopidogrel (Plavix). It also should not be combined with trazodone (used for insomnia). Talk to your doctor before using ginkgo if you are taking any type of seizure medication, as the herb may reduce the effects of the drugs. Avoid ginkgo if you are hypersensitive to mangoes, cashews, or poison ivy. Side effects of ginkgo may include mild stomach or intestinal upset.

When shopping for ginkgo, look for products that are standardized, which means they are guaranteed to contain a standard amount of active ingredients. The active ingredients in ginkgo are called flavonoids, or ginkogolides, which are believed to dilate the blood vessels and thus improve blood flow. Look for products that say "24% ginkgo flavonoids" or "24% ginkgo glycosides."

GINGER

When you were a child, did your mother give you ginger ale when you felt nauseous and dizzy after a trip in the car? If so, that's because she knew that ginger "settles the stomach." Ginger root is an herbal remedy that relieves dizziness, nausea, vomiting, and sweating that accompanies motion sickness. Its powers come from chemicals named zingiberene, gingerol, and shogoal.

To help prevent seasickness, research shows that taking 500 milligrams two hours before your trip can prevent nausea. For nausea, the suggested dosage is one 250-milligram capsule up to four times daily. You can also buy ginger tea (in teabags); drink up to three cups daily.

As a precaution, if you want to take ginger and are taking any blood-thinning medications, talk to your doctor first. This combination may result in bleeding.

VALERIAN

Many herbalists consider valerian (*Valeriana officinalis)* to be one of the most relaxing herbs available. It is sometimes used as a natural alternative to benzodiazepines (e.g., Valium), because both valerian and benzodiazepines affect the levels of a brain acid called gamma aminobutyric (GABA), which plays a role in relaxation, mood, and sleep. Valerian contains compounds that may make inactive or block the enzyme that breaks down GABA; this then allows GABA levels to increase.

For anxiety, a typical dose of valerian is 200 to 400 milligrams taken one to four times daily. You should look for products that are standardized to contain 0.8 to 1 percent valerenic acid. The calming effects of valerian are milder than those of benzodiazepines, but the occurrence of side effects is much lower. Benzodiazepines commonly cause drowsiness, especially when you first take them, as well as weakness and confusion. Valerian may cause headache or restlessness if it is taken for a prolonged period of time, but short-term use typically causes no problems.

Homeopathic Remedies

Although I personally have not utilized homeopathic remedies to treat my patients and am not a true believer in the homeopathic principles, I include this section for completeness of the complementary remedies. Homeopathy is a therapeutic approach that has been practiced for nearly 200 years, and it is becoming more and more popular in the United States. In fact, thousands of medical doctors have become certified homeopaths and offer homeopathic remedies to their patients. Some of those remedies are especially for dizziness.

Because the concept behind homeopathy is unlike that of conventional medicine, it helps to have an idea of how it works. Homeopathy is based on the concept of treating "like with like." This means that, if you take a homeopathic remedy for watery eyes and a runny nose, for example, the substance you take is one that, if taken in a larger amount and by a well person, actually causes those same symptoms. Therefore, the homeopathic remedy allium cepa (red onion) is used to treat watery eyes, runny nose, sneezing, and other cold symptoms.

The allium cepa remedy, like other homeopathic remedies, contains only a minute amount of the substance. That is based on another concept of homeopathy: potentization, or minimum dose. This concept holds that repeated dilution of a substance increases rather than decreases its healing abilities while also eliminating the risk of side effects. The more a substance is diluted, the stronger its curative powers. Thus a 6C remedy is weaker than a 12C, which is weaker than a 30C. (The "c" stands for "centesimal" and indicates how much the remedy has been diluted.) These three potencies are the ones recommended for individuals who self-treat. Consult a professional homeopath before taking more potent remedies.

In fact, even though homeopathic remedies are considered to be safe, it is best to consult a professional before taking them. Homeopathic remedies are highly individual: they are chosen to match not only each person's specific symptoms but also each person's personal characteristics and circumstances. Even if two people have the same diagnosis, they will likely receive different remedies, as different people respond differently to different substances.

Stress Reduction

It's been well proven that relaxation techniques and relieving tension can reduce or eliminate a myriad of symptoms, including dizziness, anxiety, headache, migraine, nausea, and various types of pain. Some of the most effective relaxation techniques for these symptoms include self-hypnosis, meditation, progressive relaxation, visualization, and yoga.

We'll take a brief look at each of these approaches. However, it may not matter so much which relaxation technique you choose as long as it allows you to reach the results you are seeking, because all these approaches have one thing in common: they promote relaxation and relieve stress. You may feel more comfortable practicing meditation, for example, than self-hypnosis; it is a matter of personal preference.

MEDITATION

Meditation is a practice in which you focus your mind to achieve a state of relaxation and heightened consciousness. It's been demonstrated that when people meditate, they experience a rise in natural relaxation hormones, a decrease in breathing and heart rates, and a reduction in tension, stress, and anxiety. Meditation is credited with helping people achieve feelings of calm, peace, and joy and in successfully easing dizziness, high blood pressure, aches and pains, circulation problems, breathing difficulties, and headaches.

There are two basic approaches to meditation: concentrative and mindfulness. In the former, you concentrate on something repetitive, such as a repeated word or phrase, a single object (e.g., a lit candle), or your breathing. This concentrated effort allows you to still your mind and rid it of extraneous thoughts. This is the type of meditation that was made famous in the 1970s by Herbert Benson, M.D., who conducted studies showing that concentrative meditation can decrease the heart rate and the breathing rate.

Mindfulness meditation can be likened to passive participation: you allow yourself to be aware of your thoughts, but you let them drift by without thinking about them. Instead, you simply exist in the present, letting your mind stay clear and at peace.

Many hospitals and medical centers now have meditation groups and stress reduction clinics that teach meditation. Meditation groups run by churches, support groups, and community groups are also available in many cities. If you don't care to join one of them, you can also learn meditation from audiotapes and books. (See Suggested Reading.)

PROGRESSIVE RELAXATION

This form of stress-reduction therapy helps you reach a state of deep relaxation using breathing, mental imagery, and contraction and relaxation of specific muscle groups. Some experts believe that when you tense your muscles and then relax them, you can achieve a greater degree of overall relaxation.

To practice progressive relaxation, all you need is a quiet place where you can be uninterrupted for about 15 minutes. Get comfortable: lie down or sit in a recliner that is tilted all the way back. Wear loose clothing.

- Before you begin, take several slow, deep breaths and let them out slowly: Breathe in through your nose to a count of six, hold your breath for a few seconds, then release it slowly through your mouth to a count of six.
- Close your eyes and breathe normally. Beginning with your hands, clench your fists as tight as you can. Hold the clench for five to ten seconds, then relax your hands.
- As you relax your hands, imagine all the tension in your body is escaping through your fingers and leaving you forever.
- Then clench your toes, hold, and release. Again imagine tension is leaving your body.
- Keep moving up your body to your calves, thighs, hips, pelvis, stomach, and so on.
- When you reach your head, tighten and release the different facial muscles that control movement of your mouth, eyes, nose, and forehead.

Progressive relaxation can be learned from audiotapes that will guide you through each body part and talk you through as you release tension. Check your local library or see Suggested Reading.

SELF-HYPNOSIS

Although there is little scientific research to document the effectiveness of hypnosis for the relief of vertigo, anecdotal reports seem to support it. Hypnosis, either with the guidance of a hypnotherapist or self-hypnosis, can help individuals overcome the fear-of-height vertigo or getting dizzy at heights when looking down.

Several studies have shown that hypnosis is also effective against migraine, including cases in which people use the suggestion that their head is getting cooler while their hands are getting warmer. This is essentially the same approach that can be used by people who try thermal biofeedback (see "Biofeedback" in this chapter).

VISUALIZATION

Close your eyes and picture yourself on a beautiful beach. Feel the warm breezes, inhale the aroma of tropical flowers and salt air, and listen to the call of sea gulls. If you've ever immersed yourself in a daydream that "takes you away," you've practiced visualization. During visualization, you enter a very relaxed state and focus your attention on positive scenes or images in your mind's eye. You then adjust what you see to bring about a desired result. Studies show that people have successfully used visualization to get relief from stress and pain (including migraine and arthritis), to improve blood circulation, to relieve depression, and to dispel phobias. Visualization is often used during biofeedback, but it can also be practiced alone.

A theory as to why visualization works says that people's brain activity in the cerebral cortex (the area of the brain where visual, auditory, and touch imagery are produced) is the same whether they actually experience something or they just have a vivid picture of it in their minds. This has been shown on a sophisticated scanning technique called positron emission tomography (PET). (Close your eyes for a moment and picture a lemon. Now imagine you are cutting the lemon in half and placing one half in your mouth. Is your [real] mouth puckering up?)

Thus visualization may be an effective tool for you to manage migraine accompanied by vertigo, eliminate a phobia, or deal with depression and dizziness. Visualization can be learned from books and tapes (see Suggested Reading), or you can contact instructors (see appendix C).

Yoga

The ancient practice of yoga is a method by which you can integrate and balance your body, mind, and spirit and create a calm state of being. It has been proven to reduce stress, depression, and anxiety, all of which are associated with dizziness. It also helps you improve your flexibility and strength, which are helpful in maintaining balance.

There are many different forms of yoga, but the most common ones incorporate meditation, stretching movements and postures, breathing techniques, and spiritual practice. You should consult your health-care practitioner before beginning yoga practice, and work with skilled individuals who understand the types of movements that will be most beneficial and safe for you. That's because certain movements and postures should be avoided, depending on the severity of your dizziness or balance problems. Anyone who has a balance problem, for example, should avoid head stands, shoulder stands, or back bends.

Bottom Line

Complementary therapies offer a wide variety of approaches to managing dizziness, vertigo, disequilibrium, and their associated symptoms. Many of the options discussed in this chapter can be done on your own. However, for your own safety, we recommend that you talk to your health-care providers before initiating any of these therapies.

Epilogue

The Future of Balance Disorders

From the inner ear to outer space, that's the extreme to which scientists are going to find help for people who have balance problems. Despite the significant volume of knowledge doctors and other experts have gathered so far about dizziness, vertigo, and balance disorders, they are really only just beginning to understand the complexities of these conditions. Nearly all of the treatments we have now at our disposal can relieve symptoms, but they do not cure the disorders. We don't know how to prevent debilitating conditions, such as Ménière's disease, because we don't yet know what causes them. And as our population grows increasingly older, the percentage of people who will experience age-related balance problems will grow as well.

These are the challenges that face us and just some of the reasons why experts hope they will soon discover ways to prevent vestibular disorders, as well as develop medications and procedures that will more effectively treat them. Much of this discovery process is being tackled by different organizations, institutions, and balance facilities around the country. One such organization is the National Aeronautics and Space Administration (NASA).

Value of Space Research

The weightless state of outer space is a unique and rich environment for research on balance problems. That's because disturbances to the nervous and sensory systems provoked by space travel can cause difficulties with balance, posture, and hand-eye coordination. On Earth, we have the advantage of being able to use the gravity receptors in the inner ear. In outer space, however, there is no gravity, so these receptors don't receive the signals they need to prevent balance and coordination problems. Scientists study how these functions are disturbed by space flight with the hope of gaining a better understanding of balance and coordination disorders and more effective solutions for them.

So far, information gathered from dozens of space flights have allowed scientists to study the effects of weightlessness on balance in astronauts once they returned to Earth and to apply what they learn for people on Earth who have balance problems. One advancement that has come out of these research studies is a special device that allows doctors to better test and evaluate balance disorders. The instrument helps patients regain the equilibrium and endurance they may have lost as a result of a vestibular or central nervous system disorder or a head injury.

SEVERAL HEADS ARE BETTER THAN ONE

In 1993, the NASA Appropriations Act proclaimed that NASA and the National Institutes of Health would establish a collaborative group dedicated to space-based biomedical research projects.

NASA agreed to work with groups such as the National Institute on Aging, the National Cancer Institute, the National Institute of Research Resources, and the National Institute on Deafness and Other Communication Disorders. Research is underway and will continue on Shuttle flights as well as on the International Space Station.

In 1998, a collaborative effort was launched between NASA, the National Institute on Deafness and Other Communication Disorders, and other institutes at the National Institutes of Health (NIH). These organizations joined forces to form Neurolab, a research mission that gathered information during the April and May 1998 Space Shuttle Columbia flight. Neurolab focused on the life sciences, including the balance system. One of Neurolab's goals was to study vestibular function and the physiological mechanisms that are involved in balance disorders. Special testing and monitoring systems and programs have been developed in order to conduct these studies, and it is hoped that eventually the new technology will be useful for helping people on Earth who have various balance problems.

Neurolab also provided data on the effects of weightlessness on orthostatic hypotension and other conditions that disrupt blood pressure—cardiovascular conditions which play a significant role in dizziness, balance problems, and falls on Earth and which also affect astronauts when they return from space. Scientists hope to develop treatments or preventive measures for the astronauts that will then be applicable to Earth-bound individuals as well.

NEVER TOO OLD

Much of the world held its breath in October 1998 when former astronaut John Glenn, then Senator John Glenn, age 77 years young, donned a space suit and participated in the Space Shuttle Discovery mission October 29 through November 7, 1998. Prior to that flight, NASA had gathered balance control information from much younger astronauts after they returned from space. The Discovery flight allowed scientists to collect data from a much older individual, which they hope will eventually help explain how people can recover from balance disorders they experience not only in space but here on Earth as well. They also plan to use what they learn to develop strategies to prevent injuries from falls, a significant problem especially among older individuals.

Virtual Reality

Imagine strapping on a special helmet equipped with video screens and headphones and suddenly being transported into another "reality"—a computer-generated, three-dimensional scene that unfolds right before your eyes. Welcome to the world of virtual reality, in which people are exposed to artificially created three-dimensional virtual worlds that are monitored and manipulated by a therapist.

Virtual reality has already proved successful in helping people to overcome phobias—fear of flying, heights, spiders, and so on—and to control severe pain. Now, research at various universities is focusing on using virtual reality to treat vertigo and to enhance vestibular rehabilitation therapy. One research project is called Balance NAVE (Nave Automatic Virtual Environment) and involves the use of personal computers, a battery of projectors and screens, and special goggles. Balance NAVE allows therapists to create and control varying degrees of sensory conflict, or "mixed messages," in a virtual three-dimensional environment, which assists the brain in compensation. Work with Balance NAVE is still in its early stages, but so far it is showing promise as a tool for vestibular rehabilitation therapy and balance research.

Virtual reality has even entered outer space. A new project called VOILA (Visumotor and Orientation Investigations in Long Duration Astronauts) will use virtual reality and allow scientists to study astronauts' responses to weightlessness over a three-to-five-month period. While wearing a head-mounted virtual reality display, astronauts will go through various tests—two before their flight, three during the flight, and three after the flight, to compare the effect of weightlessness on movement control. Experts believe the results of these tests could lead to new ways to evaluate balance and motor disorders on Earth and to develop new rehabilitation techniques.

VOILA incorporates some of the information collected during the 1998 Neurolab mission and builds on it. The VOILA experiments were scheduled to begin in 2003.

Be a Part of the Future

If you're someone who likes to be part of the action, you might consider enrolling in a study or clinical trial that is exploring treatment or rehabilitation options for dizziness and balance disorders. This type of research is being conducted all the time, usually at medical facilities and large universities, and plays an important role in furthering our knowledge of balance functioning. Typically, these studies don't cost participants anything except their time; some projects reimburse people for travel or even offer a small stipend. All tests and medications (if there are any) are free.

If you think you might be interested in joining a study, ask your doctor if there are any in your area that address your particular problem. You can also contact any vestibular rehabilitation centers or medical centers in your area for information. Another source is a website sponsored by the National Institutes of Health: http://clinicaltrial.gov. This website allows you to search for clinical trials in specific fields and locations and provides contact information.

If you decide to participate in a research study, make sure you understand all the procedures and what is expected of you. Before you begin to participate in a study, you will be given written information about the research, and you'll be asked to sign a consent form. Take the time to read everything that is given to you and ask questions if there is anything you don't agree with or understand. Never sign a consent form until you are comfortable with its contents. Make sure you are guaranteed that all your medical records will be held in strict confidence and that you can leave the study at your discretion.

Bottom Line

The future of treatment and prevention of dizziness and balance disorders is promising. No one can be sure whether the next discovery will come by way of outer space or a research study, but experts are confident that improvements are on the horizon. Until they get here, we hope this book has helped you get answers to your questions and, more important, effective treatment options to keep you in balance.

Appendix A

Medications

Here's a brief description of the different types of drugs used to treat dizziness and its associated symptoms. Ask your doctor or pharmacist for complete prescribing and background information on any drug you are given. You can also consult one of many consumer drug books or the *Physician's Drug Reference* for details (see Suggested Reading).

Drugs That Treat Vertigo, Dizziness, and Associated Symptoms

Drugs in this group help reduce the severity of dizziness, vertigo, and nausea once they've occurred, but they cannot prevent them, except when they are taken for motion sickness. These drugs are typically not taken for more than a few days because they can interfere with the brain's natural ability to compensate for dizziness and thus make recovery from symptoms take much longer. They also may result in dependence in some people.

ALPRAZOLAM

This sedative (Xanax) is effective against anxiety and the dizziness that can accompany it. Drowsiness and addiction are the two main side effects.

DIAZEPAM

Better known under the brand name Valium (also Diastat, Diazepam Intensol, and Dizac), this drug is a sedative that is effective against vertigo. If you take the oral form, its effects become apparent within two hours. If you receive an intravenous dose from your doctor, the effects will be immediate.

Because diazepam can cause excessive drowsiness, it should be used very cautiously in the elderly. Continuous or high use of diazepam can cause addiction, so it should be used for a short time only and under a doctor's supervision.

DIMENHYDRINATE AND DIPHENHYDRAMINE

These two antihistamines (Benadryl and Dramamine, respectively) are usually prescribed for allergies, and they are most helpful in people who experience dizziness related to allergies. Their most prominent side effect is drowsiness; dry mouth, loss of coordination, blurry vision, and dizziness can occur but are much less common.

DROPERIDOL

Droperidol (Inapsine) is a tranquilizer that is effective for acute control of vertigo and vomiting. This drug is available as an injection and is usually given in a hospital or emergency department setting.

It provides relief within 30 minutes of the injection and can last as long as 24 hours. Side effects include drowsiness and hypotension. People with liver or kidney disease should avoid this drug.

MECLIZINE

You may know this drug as Antivert (the prescription form) or as Bonine and Dramamine II (its nonprescription forms). Meclizine is an antihistamine which is most often prescribed to help prevent nausea and vomiting associated with motion sickness and which is somewhat helpful in the treatment of vertigo associated with vestibular disease. It reaches maximum effectiveness seven to nine hours after you take it; thus it doesn't provide any benefit for acute attacks of short duration. However, it's a good choice if you are taking a cruise or traveling by train, plane, or motor vehicle or if you suffer from recurrent attacks of vertigo.

The most common side effects of meclizine are blurry vision, dry mouth, drowsiness, and fatigue. People who have asthma, pulmonary disease, prostate hypertrophy, or untreated glaucoma should not take meclizine.

PROMETHAZINE

This drug (available as Anergan, Antinaus, Pentazine, Phenerzine, and Phenergan, among others) is used primarily to treat severe vertigo accompanied by nausea and vomiting, but it is also effective in suppressing dizziness. It should be used only for acute attacks and not to prevent recurrent attacks. It begins to be effective within 1 to 2 hours of ingestion, and the benefits last from 4 to 12 hours. Drowsiness is its most significant side effect.

SCOPOLAMINE

Many people choose scopolamine (Transderm Scop) when they are going on a cruise, because it is probably the most effective and convenient drug for motion sickness. It is available as a patch that dispenses the drug through the skin for three days, after which you can apply another patch.

Scopolamine helps treat mild to moderate vertigo and dizziness. It is not useful for treatment of brief episodes of vertigo because it takes four to eight hours for the drug to reach maximum effectiveness. Drowsiness and dry mouth are the most common side effects. Rarely, amnesia, urinary retention, disorientation, and hallucinations occur, and for this reason scopolamine should not be used by children or the elderly. It also should be avoided by anyone who has glaucoma or prostate enlargement.

Other Medications

These drugs are frequently used to treat Ménière's disease, migraine with vertigo, or, in the case of fluoride, otosclerosis.

• Antiemetics. Used specifically to stop nausea and vomiting and can be taken along with meclizine, scopolamine, or diphenhydramine. Two antiemetics frequently used to treat vertigo include prochlorperazine (Compazine) and metoclopramide (Maxolon, Octamide, and Reglan). Side effects can include blurry vision, drowsiness, dizziness, lightheadedness, weight gain, dry mouth, and constipation.
• Beta-blockers. Limit the tendency of blood vessels to overdilate (expand). Drugs include atenolol (Tenormin), metaprolol (Lopressor), propranolol (Inderal), nadolol (Corgard), and timolol (Blocadren). Side effects can include drowsiness; cold hands and feet; dry mouth, eyes, and skin; and dizziness.
• Calcium channel blockers. Dilate the small blood vessels of the inner ear; this improves blood flow. Drugs include nifedipine (Adalat), nimodipine (Nimotop), and verapamil (Calan). Side effects can include dizziness, lightheadedness, flushing, weakness, and diarrhea, although they are usually mild.

- Corticosteroids. Used infrequently. Some doctors prescribe short-term use of steroids for vestibular neuronitis and during the early stages of Ménière's disease to help control hearing loss. The steroids typically prescribed include prednisone (Deltasone), methylprednisolone (Medrol), or dexamethasone (Decadron). Side effects may include acne, indigestion, stomach upset, headache, insomnia, increased appetite, weight gain, dizziness, water retention, and increased tendency to bruise.

- Diuretics. Help the kidneys excrete excess fluid and are effective in relieving vertigo in migraine with vertigo. Diuretics are often prescribed along with a low-salt diet for the treatment of Ménière's disease. Three effective medications are hydrochlorothiazide/triamtrene (Dyazide), hydrochlorothiazide (Hydrodiuril), and acetazolamide (Diamox and Dazamide). Side effects can include rash, muscle cramps, weakness, dizziness, and diarrhea.

- Fluoride. Oral doses of sodium fluoride may stabilize the hearing loss that is associated with otosclerosis. The fluoride reduces the amount of bone that is absorbed, promotes the growth of new bone, and thus virtually stops any further progression of the damage. Sodium fluoride also can reduce symptoms of disequilibrium and ringing in the ears. Side effects can include rash and gastrointestinal upset.

- Gentamicin. When small doses of this antibiotic are administered directly into the inner ear of people who have Ménière's disease, it can control vertigo by reducing the function of the balance portion of the inner ear. Hearing is usually not significantly affected.

- Tricyclic antidepressants. Can be effective in controlling vertigo in patients with migraine. They include amitriptyline (Elavil), desipramine (Norpramin), doxepin (Sinequan), and nortriptyline (Pamelor). Side effects include dry mouth, dry eyes, constipation, and reduced urinary flow.

Appendix B

Other Conditions That Can Cause or Are Associated with Dizziness or Balance Disorders

- Autoimmune ear disease. An uncommon disease usually treated with corticosteroids and vestibular rehabilitation therapy
- Cogan's syndrome. Autoimmune condition characterized by dizziness, hearing loss, and eye inflammation
- Encephalitis. Viral, inflammatory disease of the brain
- Herpes zoster. Viral infection that can cause vertigo and hearing loss
- Leukemia. Blood cancer, characterized by an abnormally high level of white blood cells
- Malnutrition. Especially deficiencies of B vitamins
- Megadoses of vitamins. Especially vitamin A and niacin

- Pregnancy. Lightheadedness or dizziness which may be caused by fluctuations in hormone levels or blood pressure, or other factors
- Sickle cell anemia. An inherited condition in which people are highly susceptible to infections
- Sunstroke. Overexposure to the sun, in which the body's temperature rises to more than 107 degrees
- Temporomandibular joint disorder. Condition that affects the jaw joint and muscles
- Tuberculosis. Chronic bacterial infection, usually of the lungs, but which can invade the labyrinth

Appendix C

Resources

Organizations

Acoustic Neuroma Association
600 Peachtree Parkway, Suite 108
Cumming GA 30041-6899
1-770-205-8211
www.anausa.org

American Academy of Environmental Medicine
PO Box CN1001-8001
New Hope PA 18938
1-215-862-4544

American Academy of Otolaryngology, Head & Neck Surgery
One Prince Street
Alexandria VA 22314
1-703-836-4444
www.entnet.org

American Diabetes Association
1701 N Beauregard Street
Alexandria VA 22311
1-800-DIABETES
www.diabetes.org

American Heart Association National Center
7272 Greenville Avenue
Dallas TX 75231
1-800-AHA-USA1
www.americanheart.org

American Tinnitus Association
PO Box 5
Portland OR 97207-0005
1-503-248-9985
www.ata.org

Arthritis Foundation
PO Box 7669
Atlanta GA 30357-0669
1-800-283-7800
www.arthritis.org

Association for Applied Psychophysiology and Biofeedback
10200 West 44 Avenue, Suite 304
Wheat Ridge CO 80033
1-303-422-8436

Epilepsy Foundation of America
4351 Garden City Drive
Landover MD 20785
1-800-EFA-1000
www.efa.org

Glaucoma Research Foundation
490 Post Street, Suite 1427
San Francisco CA 94102
1-800-826-6693
www.glaucoma.org

National Coalition Against Misuse of Pesticides
701 E Street SE #200
Washington DC 20003
1-202-543-5450
www.beyondpesticides.org

National Institute of Neurological Disorders and Stroke
PO Box 5801
Bethesda MD 20824
1-800-352-9424
www.ninds.nih.gov

National Institute on Deafness and Other Communication
Disorders
31 Center Drive, MSC 2320
Bethesda MD 20892
www.nidcd.nih.gov
Contact through website.

National Mental Health Association
1021 Prince Street
Alexandria VA 22314-2971
1-800-684-7722

National Multiple Sclerosis Society
733 Third Avenue
New York NY 10017
1-800-FIGHTMS
www.nmss.org

National Neurofibromatosis Foundation
95 Pine Street, 16th Floor
New York NY 10005
1-800-323-7938
www.nf.org

National Space Biomedical Research Institute
One Baylor Plaza, NA-425
Houston TX 77030
1-713-798-7412
www.nsbri.org

National Stroke Association
9707 East Easter Lane
Englewood CO 80112
1-800-STROKES
www.stroke.org

Parkinson's Disease Foundation
710 West 168 Street
New York NY 10032
1-800-457-6676
www.pdf.org

Society for Clinical and Experimental Hypnosis
128-A Kings Park Drive
Liverpool NY 13090
www.hypnosis-research.org/hypnosis

Vestibular Disorders Association
PO Box 4467
Portland OR 97208
1-503-229-7705
www.vestibular.org

Where to Buy Nontoxic Home, Garden, and Cleaning Products

This list is representative of the many companies that provide nontoxic health and beauty products, pest control options, and cleaning supplies. You can search the Internet using key terms such as *nontoxic, natural,* and *environmentally friendly* along with terms for the specific type of product you wish to find (e.g., *beauty products* and *pest control*) for additional resources.

A+ Allergy Supply
8325 Regis Way, Los Angeles CA 90041
1-800-86-ALLER
Air purifying products, vacuum cleaners, and water purifiers

Allergy Alternative
440 Godfrey Drive, Windsor CA 95492-8036
1-800-838-1514
Air purifying products, health and personal hygiene products, nutritional supplements, and water purifiers

The Allergy Store
PO Box 2555, Sebastopol CA 95473
1-707-832-6202
Air filters and purifiers, bedding, household cleaning products, health & personal hygiene products, nutritional supplements, and water purifiers

American Environmental Health Foundation Inc.
8345 Walnut Hill Lane #200, Dallas TX 75231
1-800-428-aehf
www.aehf.com
Bedding, building materials, household cleaning products, nontoxic art supplies, health and personal hygiene products, pet care products, nutritional supplements, and water purifiers

Aubrey Organics
4419 N. Manhattan Avenue, Tampa Fl 33614
1-800-282-7394
Natural health and personal hygiene products

Biological Control of Weeds
1140 Cherry Drive, Bozeman MT 59715
1-406-586-5111
Alternative pesticide products

The Body Shop
45 Horsehill Road, Cedar Knolls NJ 07927-2003
1-800-541-2535
Natural health and personal hygiene products

Care2
Care2.com Inc
535 Middlefield Road, Suite 200
Menlo Park CA 94025
1-650-328-0198
www.care2.com/shopping
Resource for natural household products, alternative pest control products, health and beauty items, and filters

Eco Directory
www.naturalfoodsdirectory.com/
Directory of sources of organic foods, herbs, natural household products

EcoSource
PO Box 1656, Sebastopol CA 95473
1-800-274-7040
Air purifying products, building materials, cleaning products, health and personal hygiene products, pesticide alternatives, nutritional supplements, and water purifiers

Ecology Box
2260 S Main Street, Ann Arbor MI 48103
1-800-735-1371
Bedding, building materials, household cleaning products, and health and personal hygiene products

Greenpeople Directory
www.greenpeople.org/healthfood.htm
Listings of food co-ops, health food stores, and natural food stores in the United States

Karen's Nontoxic Products
1839 Dr. Jack Road, Conowingo MD 21918
1-800-527-3674
Building materials, childcare products, cleaning products, health and personal hygiene products, natural pesticide alternatives, and nutritional supplements

Living Source
7005 Woodway Drive #214, Waco TX 76712
1-817-776-4878
Air purifiers, natural household cleaning products, organic food, health and personal hygiene products, natural pesticide alternatives, nutritional supplements, and water purifiers

N.E.E.D.S.
527 Charles Avenue, Syracuse NY 13209
1-800-534-1380
Air purifying products, nutritional supplements, and water purifiers

Nontoxic Environments
9392 South Gribble Road, Canby OR 97103
1-503-266-5244
Air purifying products, building materials, heating and cool-

ing systems, health and personal hygiene products, rugs and carpets, and nutritional supplements

Organic Pest and Termite Control
PO Box 55223, Phoenix AZ 85087
1-602-923-1457
www.arizonaorganic.com

Peaceful Valley Farm Supply
PO Box 2209, Grass Valley CA 95945
1-888-784-1722
www.groworganic.com

Priorities
70 Walnut Street, Wellesley MA 02181
1-800-553-5398
Natural household cleaning products, and vacuum cleaners

Real Goods
Ukiah CA 95482-5507
1-800-762-7325
www.realgoods.com/index.cfm
Air purifiers, solar systems, and health and personal hygiene
products

Seventh Generation
Colchester VT 05446-1672
1-800-456-1177
Natural home cleaning products, health and personal
hygiene products, and building materials

Wellness, Health and Pharmaceuticals
2800 South 18 Street, Birmingham AL 35209
1-800-227-2627
Natural household cleaning products, health and personal

hygiene products, and nutritional supplements

Natural and Organic Foods

Note: Check the Yellow Pages under "Health Food" or "Organic Foods" for local listings.

Ecology Sound Farms
42126 Road 168, Orosi CA 93647
1-209-528-3816

The Green Earth
2545 Prairie Avenue, Evanston IL 60201
1-800-332-3662

Organic Consumers Association
6101 Cliff Estate Road, Little Marais, MN 55614
1-218-226-4164
www.organicconsumers.org/foodcoops.htm

Sun Organic Farm
Box 409 San Marcos CA 92079
1-888-269-9888
www.sunorganicfarm.com/Merchant2/merchant.mv

Adaptive Supplies for Safer Living

Care4U Senior Resources
www.care4u.com
Order on line.

Comfort House
1-800-359-7701

www.comforthouse.com
On line catalogue

Total Living Company
5 East Napa, Sonoma CA 95476
1-707-939-3900
www.totalliving.com

Glossary

Acoustic neuroma. A benign brain tumor that develops on the eighth cranial nerve, the nerve responsible for transmitting balance and auditory signals from the ear to the brain.

Aminoglycosides. A type of antibiotics that can damage the vestibular system.

Ampulla. The expanded or dilated ends of the semicircular canals in the inner ear. They are responsible for sensing rotation and thus are involved in balance.

Anemia. A condition in which there is a deficiency of red blood cells, which can be caused by several factors. Dizziness and disequilibrium are common symptoms of anemia.

Anxiety. A feeling of agitation, fear, or uneasiness that usually arises from anticipation of a threatening situation.

Arrhythmia. Irregular heart beat.

Audiogram. A noninvasive hearing test that measures the ability to hear sounds and the ability to understand speech.

Auditory brain stem response (ABR). A noninvasive test that measures hearing. It is often used to help detect acoustic neuromas.

Balance. A system that allows people to know where their bodies are in relation to their surroundings and to maintain a desirable position and posture. Normal balance depends on information from the inner ear, sight, and proprioceptive (sensory input such as touch and pressure)receptors.

Balance disorder. Any disruption in the labyrinth, the inner ear organ that controls balance. The labyrinth works along with the visual and muscle/skeletal systems to maintain balance.

Benign. Not malignant (cancerous). Benign tumors do not spread.

Benign paroxysmal positional vertigo. A nonmalignant (benign) condition characterized by sudden (paroxysmal) episodes of vertigo that occur when the head is placed in certain positions.

Bilateral. Pertaining to both sides of the body. Bilateral Ménière's disease affects both ears.

Biofeedback. A technique in which individuals are trained to achieve some voluntary control over certain bodily functions, such as heart beat, breathing rate, skin temperature, and brain wave rhythms.

Brain stem. The portion of the central nervous system located where the upper brain is connected to the spinal cord. The brain stem is less than 3 inches long and consists of the pons, medulla oblongata, and the nuclei of the cranial nerves. It receives signals relating to balance from the inner ear, eyes, and sensory receptors throughout the body.

Caloric testing. A portion of the electronystagmography battery of tests in which warm and/or cold air and/or water is introduced into the ear to measure vestibular functions of the horizontal semicircular canals.

Central nervous system. A body system composed of the brain and the spinal cord.

Cerebellum. Center of muscle coordination in the brain.

Cerebral atrophy. Deterioration of brain cells that can have a negative effect on equilibrium.

Cholesteatoma. An abnormal growth of skin in the ear that can cause hearing and balance problems.

Cochlea. A snail-shell-shaped structure in the inner ear that is involved in hearing.

Compensation. When talking about balance disorders, it refers to the ability of the brain to make adjustments when it receives mixed signals from various parts of the body. These adjustments result in the brain's "learning" to stop the sensation of dizziness.

Computerized dynamic posturography. A test that uses computer analysis to identify the portions of the sensory or motor systems that are contributing to balance problems. The test involves standing on a moveable platform.

Computerized tomography (CT) scan. A diagnostic method that uses x-rays and computers to provide three-dimensional images of bone and tissue.

Conductive hearing loss. Hearing loss that is caused by a malfunction in or damage to the middle or outer ear.

Cranial nerves. The 12 nerves that originate in the brain. Each cranial nerve has specific functions; the eighth cranial nerve is involved in balance and hearing.

Cupula. The sensory receptors located in the ampulla, which is responsible for balance.

Disequilibrium. The sensation of imbalance or unsteadiness.

Diuretics. Drugs that promote the excretion of urine, along with potassium and sodium. They are used to treat high blood pressure and Ménière's disease.

Dix-Hallpike test. A commonly used diagnostic test to determine whether nystagmus (abnormal eye movements) occurs when the head is placed in various positions.

Eighth cranial nerve. The cranial nerve that is critical to balance and hearing. It originates in the brain and exits through the brain stem.

Electrocardiogram (EKG). A noninvasive technique that graphs the actions of the heart.

Electroencephalogram (EEG). A noninvasive diagnostic test that records the electric activity of the brain. It is often used to diagnose seizure disorders, such as epilepsy.

Electronystagmography. A battery of tests used to diagnose the cause of dizziness and vertigo. Electrodes are positioned around the eyes to monitor eye movements while various stimuli are used.

Endolymph. Fluid contained within the labyrinth.

Endolymphatic hydrops. An abnormal accumulation of endolymph fluid within the semicircular canals and sacs of the inner ear. It can cause the symptoms of Ménière's disease.

Epley maneuver. A noninvasive treatment technique for benign paroxysmal positional vertigo in which the head is placed in various positions to induce the repositioning of otoconia (particles in the inner ear), which are causing episodes of vertigo.

Eustachian tube. A narrow tube that runs between the back of the nose to the air space in the middle ear. Opening and closing the tube, which occurs when you swallow or yawn, helps balance the air pressure between the outside and the middle ear.

Fistula. An abnormal passage or canal that runs between two spaces or organs. In the ear, it usually occurs between the middle and inner ears.

Hair cells. Sensory cells in the inner ear. These cells transform the energy of sound waves into nerve signals.

Labyrinth. The inner ear, consisting of the vestibule, cochlea, and the semicircular canals.

Labyrinthectomy. A surgical procedure in which the labyrinth is intentionally removed.

Labyrinthitis. A viral or bacterial infection or inflammation of the inner ear that can cause dizziness, temporary hearing loss, and imbalance.

Magnetic resonance imaging (MRI). A painless diagnostic technique that produces images of parts of the body. No radiation is used in this technology.

Ménière's disease. An inner ear condition that can affect both balance and hearing. Symptoms include attacks of vertigo, loss of hearing, ringing in the ears, and a feeling of fullness in the ear.

Meningitis. A bacterial or viral infection of the membranes that cover the brain and spinal cord. Dizziness is a frequent symptom.

Middle ear. The air-filled part of the ear that includes the eardrum and the ossicles, three bones involved in hearing.

Migraine headache. A recurring, often severe headache that is believed to be caused by the dilation of blood vessels that go to the brain.

Motion sickness. An inner ear condition in which individuals experience dizziness, nausea, vomiting, sweating, and general discomfort when they are in motion, usually in a moving vehicle (car, bus, plane, train, boat) or amusement park ride.

Nystagmus. Abnormal, jerky movements of the eyes. Often these movements are back and forth (horizontal), but they can be up and down or rotary.

Ophthalmologist. A physician who specializes in the medical and surgical treatment of the eyes.

Oscillopsia. An optical illusion in which you believe stationary objects are moving up and down while you are walking.

Ossicles. Three tiny bones (incus, malleus, and stapes) in the middle ear that are involved in hearing.

Otitis media. Inflammation of the middle ear that is caused by an infection.

Otoliths. Sometimes referred to as "ear rocks," otoliths are tiny crystals of calcium carbonate that reside in the inner ear. They can shift their position due to gravity, movements of the head and/or neck, or trauma.

Otosclerosis. An abnormal growth of bone that develops in the inner ear. The growth typically causes hearing loss and can affect balance as well.

Otoscope. An instrument composed of a light and magnifying lens, which allows physicians to examine the outer and middle ears.

Ototoxic drugs. Medications that can damage the balance and hearing organs in the inner ear. Examples include aminoglycoside antibiotics and high doses of aspirin.

Oval window. An oval-shaped opening between the middle and inner ears.

Perilymph. Fluid found in the inner ear.

Perilymphatic fistula. A condition in which there is leakage of fluid from the inner ear into the middle ear. The cause is sometimes associated with trauma to the head or pressure-related activities.

Presyncope. A brief feeling of faintness that passes quickly and does not result in a loss of consciousness.

Proprioceptive system. The processing system that gathers information about movement from various receptors in the body (from muscles, skin, joints, and tendons) and relays them to the central nervous system.

Pursuit system. A visual system that keeps your vision focused on an object as it moves across your field of vision.

Round window. A membrane that separates the middle and inner ears.

Saccule. A structure in the inner ear that contains otoliths.

Semicircular canals. A system of three interconnected loops in the inner ear that is responsible for balance and measuring motion.

Sensorineural hearing loss. Deafness caused by failure of the acoustic nerve.

Syncope. Fainting; loss of consciousness.

Tinnitus. Often referred to as "ringing in the ears," it can sound like ringing, roaring, buzzing, humming, or other sounds in the ears or head.

Transient ischemic attack (TIA). An event characterized by a brief episode of insufficient blood flow to the brain, which can result in dizziness, tingling, or weakness of the extremities (usually on one side of the body), vertigo, slurred speech, or blurry vision.

Vertigo. A feeling as if the world around you is whirling or revolving while you're still, or the sensation that you are whirling or revolving and your environment is still.

Vestibular system. System in the body that consists of the brain and parts of the inner ear that are involved in balance. The vestibular system is responsible for maintaining balance, posture, and the body's orientation in its environment and for regulating movement.

Suggested Reading

Academic Texts

These books are suggested for those who want to delve more deeply into the mysteries of balance disorders.

Baloh, Robert, and G. M. Halmagyi, eds. *Disorders of the Vestibular System.* New York: Oxford University Press, 1996.

Baloh, Robert W. and Vincente Honrubia. *Clinical Neurophysiology of the Vestibular System* 3d ed. New York: Oxford University Press, 2001.

Buttner, U., ed. *Vestibular Dysfunction and Its Therapy.* Munich, GER: Karger, 1999.

Canalis, Rinaldo F., and Paul R. Lambert. *The Ear: Comprehensive Otology.* Philadelphia: Lippincott Williams & Wilkins, 2000.

Furman, Joseph M., and Stephen P. Cass. *Balance Disorders: A Case-Study Approach.* Philadelphia: Davis, 1996.

Goebel, Joel. *Practical Management of the Dizzy Patient.* Philadelphia: Lippincott, Willons & Wilkins, 2001.

General Suggested Reading

Bagg, Elma, et al. *Cooking Without a Grain of Salt.* New York: Bantam, 1998.

Blakley, Brian, and Mary-Ellen Siegel. *Feeling Dizzy: Understanding and Treating Dizziness, Vertigo, and Other Balance Disorders.* New York: Macmillan, 1995.

Cargill, Marie. *Acupuncture: A Viable Medical Alternative.* Westport, CT: Praeger, 1994.

Castleman, Michael. *The Healing Herbs.* Emmaus, PA: Rodale Press, 1991.

Douglas, Bill. *The Complete Idiot's Guide to T'ai Chi and Qigong.* New York, Alpha Books, 2002.

Dworkis, Sam. *Recovery Yoga: A Practical Guide for Chronically Ill, Injured and Post-Operative People.* New York: Random House, 1997.

Fisher, Stanley. *Discovering the Power of Self-Hypnosis.* New York: HarperCollins, 1991.

Francina, Suza. *The New Yoga for People Over 50: A Comprehensive Guide for Midlife and Older Beginners.* Deerfield Beach, FL: Health Communcations, 1997.

Gawain, Shakti. *Creative Visualization Meditations.* New York: New World Library, 1997. Audiocassette.

———. *Creative Visualization: Use the Power of Your Imagination to Create What You Want In Your Life.* 25th anniversary edition. New York: New World Library, 2002.

Gazzaniga, Donald A., and Michael B. Fowler. *The No-Salt, Lowest-Sodium Cookbook.* New York: Griffin, 2002.

Graedon, Teresa, and Joe Graedon. *Dangerous Drug Interactions: How to Protect Yourself from Harmful Drug/Drug, Drug/Food, and Drug/Vitamin Combinations.* New York: St. Martin's Press, 1999.

Jahnke, Roger. *The Healing Promise of Qi: Creating Extraordinary Wellness through Qigong and Tai Chi.* New York: McGraw-Hill, 2002.

Kabat-Zinn, J. *Full Catastrophic Living: Using the Wisdom of Your Body and Mind to Face Stress, Pain, and Illness.* New York: Delacorte, 1990.

Lockie, Andrew, and William Shevin. *Family Guide to Homeopathy: Symptoms and Natural Solutions.* New York: Fireside, 1993.

Lusk, Julie, ed. *30 Scripts for Relaxation, Imagery and Inner Healing.* 2 vols. Duluth, MN: Whole Person Associates, 1992.

Medical Company Inc. *PDR Family Guide to Prescription Drugs.* Three Rivers, MI: Three Rivers Press, 2002.

Mindell, Earl. *Earl Mindell's New Herb Bible.* New York: Simon & Schuster, 2000.

Monro, Robin, et al. *Yoga for Common Ailments.* New York: Simon & Schuster, 1990.

Murray, Michael T., N.D. *The Healing Power of Herbs.* Rocklin, CA: Prima Publishing, 1991.

———. *Natural Alternatives to Over-the-Counter and Prescription Drugs.* New York: Morrow, 1994.

Rossman, Martin L., MD. *Healing Yourself: A Step-by-Step Program for Better Health through Imagery.* New York: Walker, 1987.

Starke, Rodman D., ed. *American Heart Association Low-Salt Cookbook: A Complete Guide to Reducing Sodium and Fat in the Diet.* New York: Times Books, 1995.

Weinstein, Corey, and Nancy Bruning. *Healing Homeopathic Remedies.* New York: Dell Publishing, 1996.

Winter, H. Griffith, M.D. *Complete Guide to Prescription and Nonprescription Drugs 2003.* New York: Perigee, 2002.

Index

About the Author

Dr. Jack Wazen is a neurotologist—a specialist in the management of disorders of hearing and balance. Following his residency in otolaryngology/head and neck surgery at Columbia-Presbyterian Medical Center in New York City, he completed a fellowship in otology/neurotology at the Ear Research Foundation in Sarasota, Florida. He was then recruited as Director of Otology/Neurotology in the Department of Otolaryngology/Head and Neck Surgery at Columbia University College of Physicians and Surgeons.

Dr. Wazen has spent his career in clinical care and research in the field of otology/neurotology. He has lectured on this subject at numerous institutions in the United States, as well as in Europe, China, and the Middle East, and has published many articles and book chapters. He is presently Chief of Otology/Neurotology and Medical Director of Vestibular Rehabilitation at Lenox Hill/Manhattan Eye, Ear, and Throat Hospital in New York City, and maintains his academic affiliation as associate professor of clinical otolaryngology/head and neck surgery, and neurological surgery at Columbia University College of Physicians and Surgeons. He is president of the Research Institute for Hearing and Balance Disorders and maintains a private practice in New York City.